Think
Yourself
Thin

How Psychology Can Help You Lose Weight

Think Yourself Thin

by
Dr. Frank J. Bruno

HARPER & ROW, PUBLISHERS

New York, Hagerstown, San Francisco, London

First BARNES & NOBLE BOOKS edition published 1974

ISBN· 0-06-465024-3

81 10 9 8 7 6

*To those who struggle with the
problem of unwanted fat.*

Preface

The title of this book, *Think Yourself Thin*, must have appealed to you, or you wouldn't be reading this preface now. But is it really possible? Does the title promise too much? Can you really think yourself thin?

Obviously, you can't just sit down in a comfortable chair and say to yourself: *think thin, think thin, think thin*. This would be a waste of time. The phrase *think yourself thin* is intended to imply that thought is the basic element in human freedom. We can gain control over our motives and habits by self-analysis and reflection, in a word: *thinking*.

The aim of this book is to help you think yourself thin. I believe this can best be accomplished by an understanding of psychological principles that relate to weight control. There can be no question that a clearer understanding of the psychological factors in common overweight conditions is important to all of us. Unwanted fat is quite obviously a psychological problem as well as a medical problem. This is convincingly expressed in a dictionary of psychiatry edited by J. A. Brussel and George L. Cantzlaar:

> *Overweight, psychic factors in.* While overweight can arise from fundamental organic causes such as disturbances of the pituitary, psychogenic factors are far more prominent. In the absence of organic pathology, the one and only factor responsible for overweight is overeating. Diet programs usually fail because of the subject's resistance to the curtailment of food intake due to underlying psychologic motivation.

A number of years ago these lines were written by Robert Burns:

> Oh, would some power the giftie gie us
> To see ourselves as others see us!
> It wad fram many a blunder free us
> An' foolish notion.

Burns was suggesting that we could change our behavior in a positive direction if we could see ourselves more objectively. That is one of the things that reading this book can do for you. You see yourself from the outside, so to speak. As we live our lives on a day-to-day basis, we live entirely from the inside. Psychologists call this an *internal frame of reference.* Are there any ways of getting a different frame of reference, *an external frame of reference,* on ourselves? The answer is, yes. For example, watching yourself on a television tape is one way. And this is indeed a method that some psychotherapists are experimenting with as a tool in psychotherapy. The television tape playback to a certain extent achieves what Burns was talking about in his poem. However, there are other ways of working toward an external frame of reference. As noted above, reading this book will help you see yourself more objectively. By reading about other people with weight problems, and by obtaining an insight into basic psychological principles, it becomes possible for you to put a certain distance between yourself and your own problems. You stand off from your problems as an external observer, and this helps make it possible to change your own behavior. In this way, you can start to think yourself thin.

Contents

Think Yourself Thin

Chapter 1
Your Problem

You may be anywhere from five to fifty to two hundred pounds overweight. But no matter how little or how much you are overweight, you feel you have a problem. Otherwise you would not have picked up this book. And the primary questions in your mind are: Can this book help me solve my problem? Can this book help me lose weight?

Let me answer these questions in the following manner: If you believe that the primary reasons you weigh too much are because you eat more than you should, eat the wrong foods, and eat at inappropriate times, then this book is designed to help you.

Of course, there are people who are overweight because of metabolic problems and other physiological factors. It is always wise to consult a physician and obtain his medical advice. You also want to see him for the correct diet. This book prescribes no diets. If you are anything like the average overweight person, you have tried the high-protein diet, the low-carbohydrate diet, the Mayo Clinic diet, etc. You probably can count calories and carbohydrate grams as well as an expert on nutrition.

But still you can't lose weight. Why? Obviously, your problem is that you can't stick to a diet. And this problem is psychological in nature. It is your *behavior* that is the problem. And this is exactly where psychology enters the picture. Psychology is defined as *the science of human behavior.* Consequently, it is appropriate to look to psychological knowledge for help in weight control.

I know how you feel.

I was an overweight child, an overweight adolescent, and an overweight young adult. When I entered U.C.L.A. as a junior in 1950, I weighed 245 pounds. I am five feet, ten inches tall. So you can see I was about eighty pounds overweight. I think I mark the real turning point in the solution of my problem when I took my first course in the psychology of personality. This course gave me an insight into my own behavior that I had never before possessed. I had already decided to major in psychology. And the knowledge I gained from other classes contributed to my growing self-understanding. It took me two years to lose the eighty pounds. But by the time I graduated from U.C.L.A., I was a normal weight. These events transpired almost twenty years ago, and I have never had a serious weight problem since that time.

I have been thinking about how psychology can help people lose weight ever since those days at U.C.L.A. I've looked into the psychological and psychiatric research on obesity (you will find a complete list of references in the bibliography). And I've used psychotherapy with overweight clients. I have become convinced of the value of psychology as an instrument to help the overweight person.

Allow me to illustrate. Recently a client was referred by a physician to the psychological group with which I work (The Psychological Group of San Bernardino). Let's call her Mary X. Mary was twenty-four years old, and she weighed 280 pounds. She was only five feet, two inches tall. She might have been pretty—but it was hard to see it beneath one hundred seventy pounds of ugly fat. I saw Mary regularly for six months. Psychotherapy sessions lasted one hour, and her visits were scheduled for once a week. As we discussed Mary's life, and she began soul-searching, she began to realize why she overate. A rather clear pattern of frustration and depression emerged. She had a poor relationship with her mother, she didn't respect her husband, and she couldn't cope with her too-clever, seven-year-old son. She was angry with life.

She had married before finishing high school. Yet she dreamed of going to college and becoming a grammar school teacher. Whenever she talked to her husband about these plans, he accused her of wanting to get a profession so she could divorce him.

Gradually Mary began to see her overeating for what it was: an escape from a realistic confrontation with her problems. She turned to food when she was depressed in the same way an alcoholic turns to alcohol or a drug addict turns to drugs when each of them wants to escape. The meanings that overeating had for Mary were more complex than this, of course. It is sufficient now to establish that the roots of her overweight condition were psychological in nature. Other chapters in this book present a detailed analysis of the psychological factors prevalent in common overweight conditions.

Psychotherapy helped Mary gather the strength to face her

problems more realistically. Within six months she had lost over fifty pounds, and she was well on her way to a normal weight.

HOW WILLPOWER FAILS

I often hear the lament from overweight people, "I have no willpower." Let's analyze this statement. What does it mean? First, let's analyze the word *willpower*. In classical philosophy the term *will* means your conscious desire. Plato and St. Thomas Aquinas associated the will with the conscious, reasoning part of the human soul. They called this part of the soul *the mind* as opposed to another part of the soul called the *irrational soul*. (The irrational soul was "vegetative" and the basis of growth, instinct, and appetites.) The ancient philosophers thought of *the will* as the agent of the conscious mind that makes choices. This distinction between *the mind* and the *irrational soul* was first made by Plato. It was elaborated and extended by Aquinas. It is approximately the same distinction as has been made in modern times between *the spirit* and *the flesh*. And so we have the saying, "The spirit is willing. But the flesh is weak."

Thus when an overweight person says, "I have no willpower," what he really means is this: "I have a strong conscious desire to lose weight—I often resolve to lose weight; but temptation sweeps away my best resolutions."

But this is not quite the same thing as having no willpower. The fact is that most overweight people have an ample supply of willpower. They have a very strong conscious desire to lose weight. And this by definition *is* willpower. *But they don't know how to use their willpower.*

Most overweight people use willpower in a direct confrontation with temptation. And temptation wins. But there is a way out of this dilemma. Think of yourself as a swimmer in a river with a strong current. The current is temptation or your compulsive desire to overeat. Your ability to swim is by analogy your willpower. You want to get out of the river (i.e., free yourself from your compulsion). Can you swim upstream against the current? Even if you are a very strong swimmer (i.e., have a great deal of willpower), you will soon become fatigued and be swept away by the current. What can you do? Obviously, you can use your swimming strength to reach one of the shores. By going *with* the current you eventually escape it. You have options or freedom *within* the situation.

Most overweight people waste their willpower in a futile attempt to fight temptation. Very few people can lose weight by trying to use their willpower to squelch desire. Such efforts are almost always doomed to failure. Even if they lose weight by a valiant effort of will against temptation, they almost always gain the weight back.

This book is designed to show you how to use your willpower in a constructive, creative way. Specific and practical suggestions are given that show you how to "swim with" the current of your temptations and eventually escape them. The only willpower you need is the willpower to actually *do* the things suggested in this book. If you actually try out the suggestions in this book, you will find a subtle change in your attitude toward food and your eating habits.

HOW THIS BOOK IS DIFFERENT

Although there are many books on the problem of weight control, there are very few books devoted exclusively to a discussion of the psychological aspects of the problem. Of the few books that do exist, the majority treat the problem exclusively from the psychoanalytic point of view. That is to say they rely heavily upon the concepts of *unconscious motivation* and *ego defense* as explanatory principles. These are concepts derived mainly from the father of psychoanalysis, Sigmund Freud. I also think these concepts are of value. You will find them discussed in chapters two and three.

However, the insights of certain other psychologists tend to be ignored by the psychoanalysts. The principles formulated by such psychologists as Ivan Pavlov, John Watson, Clark L. Hull, B. F. Skinner, Knight Dunlap, David Premack, and others, have been passed over in popular books on the psychology of weight control. Nevertheless, the principles formulated by these men are sound, and the principles have very specific and direct applications to the problems of the overweight person. These principles tend to be categorized in a large and important subfield of psychology called *learning theory*. To a certain extent the problem of overeating is one that involves habit formation and conditioning—in a word, *learning*. So it is fairly obvious that a complete treatment of the psychology of weight control should include a discussion of learning theory. Of course, in this book I go beyond theory and talk about specific applications. At no point is theory discussed as an abstract subject. In every case I try to illustrate theoretical formulations with concrete suggestions.

Briefly then, in this book I cover the spectrum of psychological thinking on the problem of weight control. I discuss psychoanalytic principles, but I do not limit myself to them. The book is (1) a *general psychology* of weight control, and (2) a handbook of *practical suggestions*. It is my belief that you will find the book different than any other book you have ever read on weight control. As such, I think you will find it something that can help you with your weight problem.

BASED ON EXPERIENCE

An additional way in which this book is different is that it is based on a combination of personal, counseling, and academic experience. Specifically, these are the experiences which form the foundation of the book:

1. *My own battle with weight control.* As I have already indicated in this chapter, I was overweight for many years. Although I am a professional psychologist, the problem of overeating is much more than an abstract professional question to me. I believe that my own direct experiences with the problem, plus the fact that I am a professional psychologist, have placed me in a unique position to help overweight persons.

2. *Individual psychotherapy.* Many of the insights in the present book have been drawn from my experiences working with individual overweight clients. In long personal discussions with both men and women I have become familiar with the numerous psychological patterns underlying diverse eating habits. These intimate discussions have been invaluable to me in clarifying my conceptions of what can be done to help overweight persons.

3. *Group therapy.* Some of the ideas for weight control in this book come out of my experiences with groups of overweight persons. When overweight persons have the opportunity to share their attitudes and feelings with each other, it can be very revealing. Numerous invaluable suggestions for weight control have come out of these groups. And I have incorporated these suggestions in this book.

4. *Psychology of weight control classes.* My interest in the psychology of weight control has led me to offer a course in the subject at the community college where I teach psychology. I have also taught the course through the University of California Extension Division. These classes have been

well attended, and I have been forced to clarify much of my thinking on the psychology of weight control when preparing lectures for these classes. In this book I pass on to you the things I have learned in preparing for these classes.

I can't promise you that you will become thin if you read this book. That would be an absurd guarantee. Your weight loss is in the final analysis up to you, not up to me. But I think that I can promise you that this book is an honest presentation of basic psychological principles that are involved in common weight control problems. Also, the book contains many suggestions for applying these principles to yourself.

It is difficult for me to see how the overweight person can "lift himself by his bootstraps" and attain self-control without first attaining self-understanding. This book is designed to help you on the road to self-understanding, which is the royal road to the goal of controlling your own behavior. And the key to self-understanding resides in your ability to *think* and *reflect* about your behavior. It is with this perspective that I say: *You can think yourself thin.*

Chapter 2

Unconscious Motivation

In a certain sense the compulsive eater is much like a person who has been hypnotized. A subject can be placed in a trance and given a post-hypnotic suggestion. For example, the hypnotized subject might be told that after coming out of a trance, he will fifteen minutes later have a great desire for a drink of water. The subject is brought out of the trance, and to all appearances seems quite normal. But fifteen minutes later, he will take a drink of water. If asked, "Why are you taking that drink?" he may give a variety of replies. He may say, "I don't know. I just felt thirsty." Or he may add an embellishment, a *rationalization*. "I feel thirsty because it's so hot in here. Has someone turned up the temperature?" In any event, the subject does not know the real reason for his behavior, the posthypnotic suggestion. This is an example of an unconscious motive in operation, and demonstrates that the concept of unconscious motivation is a useful one to explain certain facts of behavior.

The idea of unconscious motivation was a key concept in Freud's system of psychoanalysis. But Freud did not invent the concept. In various guises you can trace the idea of unconscious motives all the way back to Plato. However, Freud did show the world the vast importance of unconscious motives in human behavior. Freud compared the human mind to an iceberg. The tip that shows above the waterline is like the conscious thought processes. The part below the surface represents the unconscious thought processes. Thus Freud thought that most of our behavior is motivated by wishes and ideas that are obscure to us. It was, of course, the purpose of psychoanalysis to dig out these unknown wishes and ideas when they were causing trouble in everyday life.

If we translate these conceptions to the problems of the overweight person, we come up with this analysis: (1) the overweight person gives conscious reasons for eating, much like the hypnotic subject, (2) the real reasons he overeats are often obscure to him, and (3) if the real reasons can be made conscious, this may help the person lose weight. Let's now discuss these ideas in further detail.

CONSCIOUS REASONS

The conscious reasons given for overeating can be divided into two categories: (1) completely superficial answers, and (2) answers that admit to the existence of an emotional factor. Let's take up these categories one at a time.

SUPERFICIAL ANSWERS

A large number of overweight persons have almost no insight into their reasons for overeating. If you ask these people why they overeat, they will generally give you a superficial answer such as, "Oh, I don't know. I just love food I guess." I remember one overweight client, Sally K., the daughter of a physician. Her father was understandably concerned about his daughter's health. She was only seventeen years old, and she weighed over 200 pounds. In her initial interview I asked her why she thought she overate, and she answered, "I think I was born with super-sensitive taste buds. I'll bet if there was some way to measure sensitivity to taste I would come out very high. I've often thought I could make my living as a professional taster—you know, like a wine taster or a coffee taster—something like that."

"What kind of food do you particularly like?" I asked.

"Chinese food," she answered. "I really dig Chinese food."

"Interesting," I said. "Would you let me take you to lunch to a Chinese restaurant next week? It will help me evaluate your taste reactions."

She agreed, and the next week we went to lunch at a Chinese restaurant. During the meal I engaged her in a conversation about her hobby, doll-collecting, and she soon lost any self-consciousness she might have had about her eating behavior. I observed that she gobbled her food, hardly tasting it at all! Not only that, she mixed everything together, so that there was no possible discrimination between the various deliciously prepared items. While her mouth was still full with one bite of food, she would stuff in another bite. Hardly chewing, she would swill down the mouthfuls with gulps of tea. This girl was not the gourmet that she said she was. Quite the contrary! She ate like a voracious hound that hadn't seen food in a week. Whatever her reason for overeating, it certainly wasn't her stated reason: taste. This girl didn't know what it was to taste food.

I remember another client, a businessman of forty-five. When I asked him why he overate, his first answer was, "I guess I just haven't got any willpower." Yet he worked six days a week at a difficult-to-run furniture-store business, and succeeded in earning a master's degree in business education from a local state college as an evening student. Does this sound like a man with no willpower?

When I confronted him with the facts of his life as evidence against the willpower theory, he replied, "Oh, I've got plenty of willpower when it comes to business and the work for my master's degree. But I haven't got any willpower when it comes to food."

This may sound like a sensible answer to you. But it only proves to me the great capacity of human beings to deceive themselves. As far as I'm concerned, I would translate his answer into the following terms: He has a great desire to succeed in business and a great desire to succeed at school. He does not have a great desire to lose weight. Instead, he has a great desire to overeat, and he goes at it with the same intensity and "willpower" that he demonstrates in his business and educational activities.

Mrs. H. was sixty years old, and about 50 pounds overweight. I asked her why she overate, and she replied, "I don't really think I have an eating problem at all. It's just that I get weak if I don't snack frequently. I get faint, you know. And I feel that I can't do my housework. So I've got to have a bite for instant sugar in my blood."

"Can't you snack on low-calorie or low-carbohydrate foods such as carrots, celery sticks, beef jerky, or cottage cheese?" I asked.

"No, that's just the problem. I have this low blood sugar problem and I will faint dead away if I do what you say. I just don't know what to do. It's hopeless, I guess."

Mrs. H. was referred to a physician for a complete medical examination, and her endocrine functions showed no significant pathology. Here was a case of a neurasthenic reaction. The term "neurasthenia" means "weak nerves." But the nerves aren't weak. The person complains of weakness and fatigue. But the causes are psychological—not physical. So Mrs. H.'s real reason for overeating wasn't any blood sugar condition. This was merely her own fancy. And it served as a convenient excuse for her eating behavior.

It is clear to see that the reasons people give for their overeating are often very superficial. If you are not convinced by now, wait until you read the chapter titled, "Oh, My Poor Ego." In that chapter we will elaborate the concept of the ego defense mechanism, and the role this plays in obscuring the real reasons for overeating.

EMOTIONAL FACTOR ANSWERS

The existence of an emotional factor in common overeating has been so popularized in the women's magazines and other places that a great many overeaters are ready to concede that their problem has emotional roots. I recently asked a group of overweight women to write out a short answer to the question: Why do you overeat? Over one-half of the replies made some reference to an emotional problem. Here are some examples:

"I eat because it consoles my inferiority complex. I also drink too much and take pills that tend to make me retain liquids."

"I am a nervous eater. I eat when I am insecure, unhappy, displeased, and anxious."

"When I become nervous or overtired the *only* thing that helps is a slice of bread with *lots* of butter."

"I overeat when I'm upset usually. And I also tell myself it will give me energy if I'm feeling tired."

15

"I use food as a crutch. Also—when I am depressed, it seems much more difficult to lose the weight."

"I know that I overeat. But I really don't know why. It's mostly an emotional problem—but I'm not sure exactly how."

"Frustration and rejection cause me to overeat. I've never had a very favorable self-image."

"I overeat primarily because I'm overweight and I guess it's the way I cope with it—quite a paradox!"

"I overeat because I get nervous or upset at myself."

"I don't know why I overeat. I think I am bored."

"I overeat because I am a nervous individual who takes out my frustrations, disappointments, fears, anger, boredom, and anxiety through my eating habits."

"I'm very insecure a great deal of the time. I find myself eating for comfort—feeling deprived and thus turn to food. Food is passive, and you don't have to deal with it! Anxiety plays a great havoc on my dieting."

In the above answers we can see a willingness on the part of many overweight persons to concede the point, that an emotional factor is involved in overeating. This is an important first step. But, of course, it is not enough. Key words are used such as inferiority, insecurity, frustration, anxiety, and boredom to explain the overeating behavior. But, unfortunately, these are just words. They are empty abstractions unless these deeper questions are answered: Why are you insecure? What are the frustrations in your life? What are the roots of your anxiety? These questions bring us directly to the concept of unconscious motivation. Feelings of inferiority, insecurity, frustration, and anxiety are manifestations of deeper problems that are often obscure, or at best half-understood. The following discussion attempts to clarify the role of unconscious motives in compulsive overeating.

UNCONSCIOUS REASONS FOR OVEREATING

What, then, are some of the unconscious reasons for over-eating? Before going into detail, let's point out the general principle that operates in unconscious motivation. An unconscious motive is a wish or a desire that is distasteful on a conscious level. It is probably a motive that we find offensive to our self-concept, and consequently we *repress* it. *Repression* is a term coined by Freud to describe an unconscious process by which unpleasant or threatening ideas are shoved out of our consciousness. Of course, repression is seldom a complete solution to our problems, and we find repressed ideas showing up again and again in dreams, slips of the tongue, and psychosomatic symptoms. This is one way of looking at the overweight person. Obesity can be seen as a psychosomatic expression of a repressed conflict.

OBESITY AS A SEXUAL DEFENSE

Mrs. Y. was a thirty-five-year-old homemaker, the mother of four children. Her husband was a successful general building contractor. Her tastes were artistic—her hobby was writing poetry. His tastes were those of the outdoor man. He went on hunting trips and had a gun collection. His language was rough and filled with four-letter words. He was a hard drinker, often drinking himself into a stupor on evenings when he was home. He worked long hours at his job, and provided a high income for the household. But Mrs. Y. bitterly resented his drinking and his lack of comprehension of her poetry. Whenever she showed a poem to her husband, he would read it quickly, and make some flip remark such as, "Another candidate for the wastebasket." Or, "How many rejection slips do you think you'll collect on this one before you give up?"

In the past five years Mrs. Y. had gone from a trim 125

pounds to 195 pounds. She was puzzled by her problem, and came up with various conscious reasons for her overweight condition. Her main explanation revolved around her thyroid gland, which she described as "sluggish." Her physician referred her for psychotherapy. An old general practicioner, he was able to discern that perhaps the roots of Mrs. Y.'s problem could be traced back to discontent with her marriage.

In psychotherapy, Mrs. Y.'s dissatisfaction with her husband became transparent. Within a few sessions she was going into great detail about the real and imagined injuries he had inflicted on her. It was also revealed that Mr. Y. hunted more than wild game. His "hunting trips" were often spent in the company of prostitutes. He and his companions would rent a mountain lodge for a weekend, and arrangements would be made with call girls to spend a night with "the boys." In the early years of his marriage Mr. Y. had made some pretense of concealment. But eventually he disclosed his behavior to Mrs. Y. Mrs. Y. was a regular churchgoer and prided herself on being a decent Christian woman. She was, understandably, shocked by her husband's escapades. She was also deeply hurt. But he brushed her off with references to the "European system." He explained in Europe it was the convention for successful businessmen to have mistresses and relationships with prostitutes. He expressed his belief in the double standard: Men were sexually free, but their wives were meant to be faithful and keep the home together. It appeared that Mr. Y. still retained the somewhat antiquated view that women were chattel, an item of personal property belonging to the man, something like his bank account or his car.

What unconscious motives were discovered in psychotherapy? Although Mrs. Y. was aware of her bitterness and hostility toward Mr. Y., she was not aware of the magnitude of her feelings. Nor did she clearly perceive how her feelings related to her overeating problem. As she gained confidence with the therapist, she was able to reveal the presence of sexual fantasies that plagued her on a conscious level. She would see a man walking in the street and wonder what he would look like in the nude. Or she would be talking to a shoe salesman and wonder what his lips would feel like during a kiss. It was extremely embarrassing for her to reveal these thoughts, and she was barely in touch with them. As soon as they occurred to her, she fought against them and banished them from consciousness. So she experienced them as only passing fancies that flitted across her mind. Nevertheless, she was extremely guilty about having them at all.

She reported a very vivid dream. She had seen herself sitting in the nude astride a long black train engine. She was a giant astride the engine, riding it like a horse. The engine was hurtling through the night in a thick forest. On the side of the engine in bold capitals there appeared the letters *S. E.*

Free association to the elements of the dream revealed that the train engine was a symbol for the male phallus. Riding the engine symbolized sexual intercourse. The night and the thick forest symbolized the female's vagina and its interior. All of this was fairly obvious. But the letters *S. E.* were something of a puzzle. At first all she could think of was "Southern Electric." But then it finally hit her, and she blurted out, "Of course! The letters *S. E.* stand for *Someone Else*. I want to have sexual relations with someone else. I want to do the kinds of things my husband is doing!"

Gradually it became apparent to her that one of the main psychological meanings to her obesity was that it was a form of defense against her repressed sexual desires. As long as she was fat and physically unattractive, what man would want her? She was protected against her own impulses. Consequently, she felt tense and anxious whenever she began to lose weight. Only by remaining obese could she maintain a sense of self-control and mental calm.

In spite of her hostility toward her husband, Mrs. Y. had no intention of breaking up her marriage. She wanted to stay married to Mr. Y., be his wife, and preserve what home life they had. She ultimately realized that the only thing she had to fear about her sexual impulses was the fear itself. She was not going to act on her impulses. Her moral code made this impossible. And she had a firm reality orientation which made continued self-control quite feasible. (This is the concept of *ego strength*. Persons with high ego strength can cope with a stiff dose of reality, and adapt to it in a practical manner.) It was now possible for Mrs. Y. to lose weight without triggering a storehouse of repressed anxieties. As Mrs. Y. became both more attractive and more pleasant to live with, something strange began to happen to Mr. Y.'s behavior. He spontaneously began drinking less and going on fewer of his hunting trips. He conceded to his wife that maybe there was something to psychology (he had been very critical of his wife's decision to see a psychotherapist), and he made an appointment with the therapist to tell his side of the story. As of this writing, the Y.s are involved in family therapy counseling, and they are working jointly to improve their relationship.

Here is an example of another situation in which the patient used obesity as a defense against sexual impulses. Miss G. was twenty-two years old, lived with her parents, and worked as a clerk in a small office. She was more than one hundred pounds overweight the first time I saw her. After several sessions she revealed that she had been seduced twice. The first seduction took place in the back seat of a car when she was seventeen. The seducer was a fellow she had met on a blind date. He was stationed at a nearby army camp, an overseas replacement depot, and was just passing through the small town in which Miss G. lived. His approach was very rough, very direct, and she capitulated almost immediately. The second seduction took place when she was nineteen. The circumstances were similar in certain ways. The seducer was a married man, had no personal interest in Miss G. as a human being, and achieved his seduction by a brash, straightforward approach. It was shortly after the second seduction that she began to gain weight. Conversations with Miss G. made it clear that one of the primary reasons underlying her obesity was that it made further seductions unlikely. She showed me a photograph of herself at one-hundred twenty pounds when she was nineteen, and it would be understandable why she was a target for seduction. But at her present weight of 220 pounds few men would be interested. Her obesity was a kind of avoidance behavior. She was protected against her own impulses by the clownlike appearance she presented to men.

Miss G. had received a very strict Christian training, and she felt very guilty about the seductions. She also had problems in relating to men as human beings. She had never formed a sound relationship with her father, and she transferred much of her hostility toward him to men in general. She let herself be seduced easily, primarily because she felt so inadequate as a female. The moment a man made a direct approach she melted. This was as if the man was saying, "Yes. You are feminine. You are desirable." She was terribly confused about her feminine role in life, her relationship with her father, and her relationship to men in general. All of this had to be dealt with in a meaningful manner before she could begin to lose weight successfully.

PASSIVE AGGRESSION

Another unconscious motive that may underly certain cases of obesity is the wish to express hostility. Let's return to the case of Mrs. Y. She was shocked and hurt by the fact that Mr. Y. cavorted with prostitutes. However, she found it difficult to express hostility directly. If she began to tell him how she felt, she would begin screaming and yelling and lose all self-control. She hated herself when she did this, and she knew it made her relationship with her husband worse. Her character pattern took on what psychologists call a *passive-aggressive* structure. That is to say she was passive and accepting on the surface. She tried to speak sweetly to her husband and maintain a false front that everything was all right. But underneath this facade she was fuming. One way of expressing this hostility was to become fat. It's rather obvious that most husbands hate to see their wives get fat. Consequently, when the husband gets "uptight" about this, makes snide remarks, and in general is displeased, the wife is getting out of him exactly what she wants. (Obviously, this can also work the same way with overweight husbands.) Mrs. Y. was telling her husband with her obesity, "You are displeased with me? Well, fine, that's just what you deserve. Because I'm plenty displeased with you too!"

This passive-aggressive hostility pattern is a common one in cases of obesity during childhood. The overweight child may be punishing his parents. When the parents nag him about food, act uncomfortable because of his obesity, this only makes matters worse. This is exactly the kind of payoff the child is looking for. He cannot express hostility in adequate ways, and the signs of discomfort from his parents are indicators that his passive-aggressive strategy is working. Tommy R. was such a child. He was in every way the "model child." He received straight A's in school, practiced the violin diligently every day, was permitted by his parents to play only with "nice" children, faithfully went to Sunday school, was a delight to his teachers because of his obedience and good manners, and never uttered an obscenity. By the time Tommy reached the age of fourteen his parents were distraught. He weighed 190 pounds. The normal weight for his age and height was 110 pounds. His parents couldn't understand it. They were sure his problem wasn't psychological because they "gave him everything." And he didn't overeat. Why he ate regular meals three times a day and that was it. But his parents didn't see the candy and between-meal snacks Tommy consumed. When medical treatment alone failed, Tommy was referred to a psychotherapist. A case such as this one requires working with the parents as well as the child before progress can be made. The parents have to be helped to see that the child's problem is largely a result of their attitudes and their behavior.

UNDERLYING DEPRESSION

Another unconscious factor that may operate in a great number of cases of obesity is the existence of underlying depression. The well-known cheerfulness of the overweight person is often a defense—a denial of the existence of depression. The overeating behavior itself may be a way of soothing oneself when one is depressed.

Let's return once again to the case of Mrs. Y. because it presents in an almost classical manner the elements we are discussing. Her case relates to a famous hypothesis in psychology called the *frustration-aggression hypothesis.* The hypothesis was proposed by Neal Miller and John Dollard of Yale University. The hypothesis suggests that there is an invariant relationship between frustration and aggression. Frustrate an organism and it gets mad. What happens under these circumstances? The psychological pattern looks something like this: (1) frustration——→aggression, (2) aggression unexpressed——→depression. So it is not difficult to comprehend the psychodynamics of Mrs. Y.'s depression. And it is not too difficult to see how this depression was a complicating factor in her overeating problem. Mrs. Y. was understandably frustrated and angry because of her husband's behavior. But much of this anger was unconscious—she repressed it because she couldn't deal with it.

FEELINGS OF INADEQUACY OR FAILURE

An unconscious idea that can play a role in obesity is the thought, "I'm unimportant. I'm nobody." One of the fathers of clinical psychology, Alfred Adler, coined the term *inferiority complex* to describe this feeling. I recall in particular the case of Sammy W. Sammy had a very mediocre job in a printing shop. His wife constantly berated him about their poor standard of living. He wanted to quit his job, take his small savings, and open a roadside doughnut shop. He was sure he could make a go of this business. His wife constantly resisted this "silly dream," and Sammy never did try out his business ideas. At parties Sammy was always the life of the party. He came prepared to do the entertaining. He used to buy prepared items at joke stores. For example, he would enter the party wearing a funny wig, a set of giant glasses, or smoking an enormous cigar. He always made the "grand entrance," arriving a little late so everybody could have a good laugh. He learned how to do imitations of fat comedians, and his favorite imitation was to act out the role of Ralph Kramden in Jackie Gleason's "The Honeymooners." In particular he liked to do the part where Ralph shakes his fist at Alice and says, "One of these days!" It doesn't take a psychologist to see the way in which he was utilizing this aspect of his clownlike behavior to express hostility toward his wife.

But one of the main psychological meanings of his obesity was his desire to compensate for his sense of unimportance. On an unconscious level there was the nagging thought, "I'm unimportant. I'm nobody. I'm a small man." And so his conscious compensation for this thought was to become a "big man." Sometimes this can work out fairly well. For example, the hard-driving businessman may be compensating for an identical thought. His personal inadequacies drive him to prove that he can be a "big man" in the business world. This may be a fairly successful way of compensating for unconsciously low self-esteem. Unfortunately, there may also be psychosomatic side effects such as ulcers and malignant hypertension. In Sammy's case, he was blocked from acting on his business ideas. So he resorted to the pitifully inadequate behavior of playing the clown to his friends.

Playing the clown may be all right as a temporary psychological crutch. But when it becomes a way of life that lasts year after year, it begins to wear thin. And often the person begins to see through his own behavior. This is what happened in Sammy's case. Little by little his defenses began to fail him, and he became more and more consciously aware of his sense of unimportance. His wife gave him the final rejection by initiating a divorce action. A few years later he was admitted to a state mental hospital with the diagnosis of *involutional melancholia*. Involutional melancholia is a form of mental illness characterized by extreme depression and lack of interest in life.

He no longer used obesity or clowning as a defense against reality. Instead, he sat for hours in front of the ward television set staring blankly. A man of medium height, he had attained 280 pounds at his maximum weight. Now he seemed to swim in his hospital robe, and the formerly full flesh appeared to hang on his bones.

In initial psychotherapeutic interviews, he would confess his depression completely. "I'm no good. I'm worthless. I never made any money. My wife hates me. My kids hate me. I wasn't a good father. I wasn't a good husband. I never did anything. I'll never do anything. What's the use? Why go on? I don't care about anything anymore." As you can see from the quotation, he was not out of touch with reality. He knew who he was, where he was, and why he was in the mental hospital. But he had what the philosopher Soren Kierkegaard called "the sickness unto death." His existence was meaningless—empty. He couldn't dream, plan, or hope for a better future.

There is no simple panacea for a condition such as Sammy's. You can't talk him out of his depression. But little by little his depression began to lift. He began to learn a new trade in the hospital: cabinet making. He found it very satisfactory to work with his hands. Also, in group psychotherapy he found out that he could be liked and accepted for himself without acting the role of the clown. Whenever he tried out his old clownlike antics on the group they pounced on him, gave him a stiff dose of reality, and told him to "cut it out." One of the members of his psychotherapy group, a woman alcoholic, took a friendly interest in Sammy. They took walks about the hospital grounds together, and chatted at length about their shattered lives and how they might rebuild them. There was a touch of romantic interest here. But to my knowledge neither of them took it very seriously. Nevertheless, the mere fact that he could have an intimate relationship with another human being—and a woman at that—did Sammy a great deal of good. In six months he was ready to be released from the hospital and make a new start in the world outside.

Very few cases in which obesity is a defense against inferiority feelings would have effects as serious as those described in Sammy's case. But Sammy's story is a dramatic illustration of the role that feelings of failure can play in overeating behavior.

THE AVOIDANCE OF THREAT

Paradoxically, overeating can be a way of avoiding people as well as a way of seeking their attention—as it was in

Sammy's case. A girl who lacks confidence in her basic appeal as a human being may use obesity as a defense against this self-knowledge. Such was the case of June Q., a seventeen-year-old high school student. June had a broad, freckled face, prominent upper teeth badly in need of orthodontic work, and a childish-sounding lisp. Boys had no interest in her, and she said to me that she had no interest in boys. She thought boys "were silly." Of course, this was not an expression of her true feeling. She was only kidding herself. She wanted boys to be interested in her, but she was deeply unsure of herself. On an unconscious level, she felt that if she lost weight she would still be unattractive to boys. This way, she could think to herself, "The reason boys don't ask me out is because I'm fat." But if she lost weight, and if boys still didn't ask her out, then she would have to face the unpleasant fact that she wasn't very attractive even at a normal weight. Her fear of rejection worked to keep her fat.

June's miserable self-image was only partly grounded in reality. Many of her feelings of low self-esteem stemmed from her family situation. Her mother was also obese. In addition she was divorced and a confused and inadequate person. (Her mother was also being treated by a psychotherapist.) June's treatment involved a number of approaches. Orthodontic work corrected the problem with her teeth. A speech therapist helped her correct her lisp. As she gathered insight and ego strength in psychotherapy, she was placed in a teen-age charm course that helped to give her poise and confidence. She learned how to groom herself to her best advantage. She learned some of the tricks of small talk and polite conversation that a girl can use to help out a boy when he is dating a girl for the first time. (Boys feel inadequate and flounder too!) By the time she was a high school senior, she was asked to the senior prom by a boy she found to be very acceptable.

June was not and never will be a great beauty. She is,

however, not an unattractive person. She is at least as attractive as the hypothetical average girl. Have you ever watched one of the broadcasts of a national beauty contest for teenage girls? I am always surprised by how basically plain many of the girls are. But they know how to use their assets to their best advantage. I have known a number of girls who are fundamentally quite average in appearance. But their make-up, hair-do, and personality easily compensate for any deficiencies they may have.

THE FEAR OF THE UNKNOWN

One of the overall motives that operates in almost all cases of obesity is the fear of the unknown. The overweight person is to some extent afraid of the new body image that will result when weight is lost. The longer a person has been overweight, the more this is a problem. The concept of a "new you" can be very anxiety-arousing. This thought may run through your head: "If I'm going to become a new me, what will happen to the me I am now?" On an unconscious level, some people feel that they are dying when they lose weight. After all, we identify with our present body image, no matter how unsatisfactory it may be. It offers a certain sense of security, a certain predictable state of affairs. We cling to it in the same way that Linus clings to his blanket. Looking at Linus, an outsider feels, "Why can't the child just get rid of that miserable blanket?" In much the same way an outsider looks at an overweight person eating an ice cream sundae in a coffee shop, and thinks, "How disgusting. Why can't that person give up those indulgences?" The outsider doesn't realize that just that morning the overweight person being watched got on the scale, saw that two pounds had been lost after three days of strict dieting, and this weight loss triggered a wave of latent anxiety. The eating of the ice cream sundae represents a flight from anxiety.

The psychologist Erich Fromm wrote a book called *Escape*

From Freedom in which he postulated that human beings find uncertainty intolerable. The ambiguity and uncertainty that comes from freedom creates anxiety. And so they "flee from freedom" into a situation that seems to offer definite answers. (In Fromm's book the hypothesis was used to explain the rise of Hitler as a dictator in Nazi Germany.) The principle is very general, and applies to many situations. It is illustrated by the famous Rorschach inkblot test. The subject is shown inkblots that are ambiguous and without any definite form or structure. However, in only a few seconds most people "make something" out of the blots. We almost have to make something out of them. We can't tolerate that vague blob of nothingness. Of course, what we see in the blots is a reflection of ourselves—of our unconscious motivational structure.

The human being's intolerance of ambiguity is reflected by the structuring of leisure time. When people have a day off or a holiday they are seldom content to relax and just do nothing. Something must be planned for the day. It's the "What are we going to do today?" syndrome. As soon as the plan is made—a trip to the zoo, a drive to the beach—then the plan becomes a little god and the whole family rushes around in order to make the plan come true in accordance with the time schedule (e.g., "we'll be on our way by 10:00 A.M., and we should arrive at the zoo for lunch by 12:00 P.M., etc.").

In much the same way, many overweight persons prefer the known structure of their lives when they are overweight, than to have to face the ambiguity and uncertainty that arises when they begin to lose weight. The unconscious resistance to a "new self" can be tremendous. I remember one patient who was about fifty pounds overweight. I asked her to have a fantasy in which she was standing in front of the mirror in a bathing suit at her normal weight. She was to describe what she saw. The patient said, "I've got a terrific body—like Raquel Welch. The image is very clear." It should be pointed out that this was highly unrealistic, and was a form of denial in itself. The patient was five feet two inches tall, and had been overweight for more than ten years. She continued, "But I can't see my face. It's just a blank." She was completely unable to see herself at a normal weight. She couldn't identify her head (i.e., her ego) with her body. She was almost denying the possibility of ever attaining a normal weight. The example clearly illustrates the great resistance that some persons offer to weight loss. Her "new you" was an impossible Raquel Welch with which she could not identify. The unrealistic Raquel Welch image was a way of saying, "This is the kind of body I'd like to have in my dream of dreams. I'll never have what I want, and so what's the use of trying at all?" In this patient's case quite a bit of time was spent with her on attaining a realistic and nonthreatening body image toward which she could work without anxiety.

WHAT CAN YOU DO ABOUT IT?

If you are suffering from all of these dark, deep unconscious motives, isn't the situation quite hopeless? Well, for one thing, the purpose of this chapter was to take a hard look at unconscious motives, bring them out into the open, and remove some of the darkness and depth from them. Once unconscious motives are made conscious, they are no longer, by definition, unconscious motives. They become conscious motives, and you can deal with them.

Although in theory almost any kind of motive can be the unconscious source of overeating, in fact the prime unconscious motives tend to fall in a few categories. These have been surveyed in this chapter. In brief, they are:

1. Repressed sexual desires resulting in unconscious sexual conflict.

2. Repressed hostility—obesity can be a form of passive aggression.
3. A defense against underlying depression arising from life's frustrations.
4. A compensation for feelings of inferiority (i.e., low self-worth, low self-esteem, poor self-concept, etc.).
5. A way of avoiding threatening and unpredictable life situations.
6. Resistance to a new body image. The "new you" is unfamiliar and threatening to the present self.

Ideally, every overweight person with a chronic problem should first see a physician. If the physician rules out the existence of constitutional factors, then the overweight person should seek adequate psychotherapy. Adequate psychotherapy usually consists of the services of a trained psychologist or psychiatrist. However, I'm also aware of the fact that most overweight persons won't do this. They buy and read books such as this one as a do-it-yourself operation. I believe in do-it-yourself too. I've seen people read books, get insights, and help themselves. It's happened to me. However, I would say that if you read books, try to lose weight for six months or one year, and are still overweight, you should seek professional aid.

Now, to be more specific, can you analyze yourself? Can you get insight into your own unconscious motives without professional help? The answer is both yes and no. I doubt that you can gain the depth of insight by self-analysis that you could get from psychotherapy. However, a number of people have attempted self-analysis, including Freud. An excellent book on this subject is *Self-Analysis* by Karen Horney. It appears that some people can grow in self-understanding by asking themselves the right questions and following certain procedures.

What are the "right" questions? What are the "certain procedures"? You could start by converting each of the prime unconscious motives for overeating into a question:

1. Do I have repressed sexual desires? What are they? Do I have unconscious sexual conflicts? What can I realistically do about these conflicts?
2. Is my obesity a form of repressed hostility? Do I use it as a form of passive-aggression? How might I express aggression in a more effective manner?
3. What frustrates me? Am I depressed because of these frustrations? Am I bored with my spouse, mad at my children, tired of my job, or disappointed in myself? What can I do to change the situation?
4. Is overeating a way of compensating for feelings of inferiority? How can I improve my self-concept? Am I inferior or do I just feel inferior? How can I act on my best capacities to shake myself out of the doldrums?
5. Do I use my overweight condition as a way of avoiding threatening and unpredictable life situations? Are my feelings rational? What would happen if I got involved in these situations? Is my anxiety just a fear of fear?
6. Am I resisting a new body image? Do I feel that substantial weight loss is a kind of death of the present self? Why do I feel this way? What can I do to overcome this feeling? If I lose weight gradually rather than abruptly, will this help me deal with a new body image?

Write out an answer to each of these questions in the greatest detail you can manage. This procedure may give you quite a bit of insight into your own motivational structure. Just writing something out helps you think more clearly about it.

I think this procedure of writing out answers is a fairly straightforward one, and can be very helpful. One way of thinking about unconscious motives is just to say that they are motives that are obscure and half-understood. As soon as you see the motive in yourself and understand it, you often have the very interesting experience of feeling that it was never unconscious in the first place. It was always there—a part of your personality structure. And of course it was. There are things about ourselves, that in a sense, we always knew, but just didn't take the time or thought to put into words.

The first time you write out answers to the questions, the answers may be "thin" and seem inadequate to you. But don't be discouraged. The attempt itself will set up a growth process in you. Try answering the questions again in a week without any reference to the first answers. Then try again a week later. You might do this once a week for several months. The insight you acquire might surprise you.

What about deep-probing techniques? Nowadays a great many amateurs try self-hypnosis, or attempt to hypnotize each other. Still others take powerful drugs such as LSD and talk to their friends in their drugged state hoping to "blow their minds" and get at their "hang-ups" or unconscious motives. There are cults of untrained amateurs who try to practice variants of psychoanalysis on each other. My own reaction to these procedures is that they are too powerful and too dangerous to be employed without professional guidance. This is not just an attempt on the part of a psychologist to keep unconscious motivation as the private jurisdiction of the professional high priests of psychotherapy. On the contrary, there is a very real danger in digging too deeply, too fast, into a person's unconscious motivational structure. If you have repressions, don't forget that there are reasons for them. Unlocking a great many unconscious motives at one time may result in a flood of material that cannot be tolerated by the ego.

However, I am *not* suggesting that you should not try to achieve self-understanding. Socrates' famous dictum, "Know thyself," is still good advice. But I am suggesting that you attempt to know yourself by the more straightforward means of intelligent, wide-awake clear thinking. There is no such thing as instant enlightenment. You have to work at it.

The purpose of this book is to help you obtain insight with your eyes wide open. Your entire life should be a voyage in which part of your travels involve self-exploration. This is one of the reasons people read psychology, philosophy, novels, and the Scriptures. They seek understanding and insight into human behavior. But we don't need drugs or hypnosis to achieve this goal. We need alert intelligence and clear thinking.

Chapter 3

Oh, My Poor Ego!

What is the human ego? The human ego is the *I*, the *self*, our sense of being a living, breathing, individual human being. This *I* wants to think well of itself. It prefers high self-esteem rather than low self-esteem. Thus when a message comes in from the outside world that produces in the ego a sensation of low self-esteem, the ego immediately retaliates with a defense. Think of the ego as the center of a medieval fortress. Around the fortress are high walls, moats, and other structures designed to keep hostile forces away. And there are archers high on the castle walls. They will shoot down attackers. Your ego is something like this. It doesn't particularly like to receive negative information from the outside. Negative information, information that lowers self-esteem, is the "enemy." Of course, persons who have high self-esteem or "ego strength," do not have such a great concern about negative information. Because they feel strong within themselves, they can permit a certain amount of negative information to penetrate their defenses, and in the long run can take advantage of this information to improve their whole personality. To extend our analogy of the medieval fortress, think of the captain of the guard of the fortress as so touchy that he shoots down willy-nilly anyone who approaches the fortress without first assessing if it is friend or foe. The person with a weak ego is something like that. Try to help him, give him good advice, and he is immediately on the defensive. Psychologists speak of *ego defense mechanisms.* These mechanisms are designed to protect the tender ego in a semi-automatic fashion. They "kick in" to operation without conscious control.

No one is suggesting that you try to get rid of your ego defense mechanisms. In the first place, this is next to impossible. Our ego defense mechanisms are so well entrenched, so much a part of our character, that their complete removal is both difficult and undesirable. We need our ego defenses. They keep us sane and functioning during times of stress. By providing a buffer between us and reality, they help make the "slings and arrows of outrageous fortune" more acceptable to us.

However, it is possible to moderate the effect of the ego defense mechanisms by an act of reflection. Sometimes we do ourselves a disservice when we refuse a message from the outside. For example, it can sometimes help to say to yourself, "Now, am I rationalizing—or is this something I really believe?"

In this chapter we will discuss some of the key ego defense mechanisms and how they relate to the problem of weight control.

RATIONALIZATION

Rationalization is one of the oldest and most well-recognized of the ego defense mechanisms. It was recognized by Aesop who wrote the famous fable of the fox who couldn't reach a bunch of grapes high on a vine. When the fox said, "Oh, well. They're probably sour anyway," this was a classic case of rationalization.

A student receives an F on an examination. He hates to think of himself as a poor student, or to admit to himself that he didn't put enough effort into preparing for the examination. If he is a student with many doubts about his competence, then rationalization provides an "easy out" for the moment. He says to himself, "That was really a stupid exam. What ridiculous questions. They were unfair and poorly worded. No wonder I got an F."

Rationalization is a procedure by which you give yourself "good-sounding" reasons instead of "real reasons" for your failures, transgressions, and shortcomings as a person.

(I suppose that a fox with a really strong ego would have said, "I would really like to have had those grapes. They *did* look sweet. It is unfortunate that they're out of my reach." This kind of thinking might have put him well on the way to inventing the ladder!)

Now let's apply some of this to the problem of overeating. Mary K. is out shopping with two of her girl friends at one of the new air-conditioned shopping centers with an enclosed mall. It is a pleasant way to spend a Saturday afternoon. The girls have spent several hours going in and out of the shops and department stores. One of the girls suggests that they stop in at an ice cream parlor for refreshments. Mary K., who is supposedly dieting, orders a double-scoop hot fudge sundae. What does she say to herself? Her thoughts run something like this: "Oh, well, it won't hurt just this one time. After all it's been a long afternoon, my feet hurt, and I used up a lot of energy walking. My blood sugar is probably low, and I need a lift. Maybe I'll skip breakfast tomorrow morning." These thoughts which come and go in an instant are examples of rationalizing statements. She is giving herself "good reasons" for her behavior instead of real reasons. If she were being realistic, she would say to herself, "This social situation is just providing me with a convenient excuse for going off my diet. The laws of nature aren't suddenly suspended because I'm out with my friends on a Saturday afternoon. The calories in a hot fudge sundae don't know I'm out shopping and that I want to suspend the rules."

Social situations in general offer many opportunities to rationalize your behavior. Here's what one patient said to me recently: "I went off my diet over the weekend. It was my nephew's birthday, and my sister-in-law would have been offended if I didn't have a piece of the birthday cake she baked." Is this a real reason or an example of rationalization? I think it's another example of rationalization. How offended would the sister-in-law have really been? If the sister-in-law has your best interests at heart, wouldn't she rather see you lose weight than remain overweight? And if she doesn't have your best interests at heart, then who cares if you offend her?

The same is true of hostesses who press food on you. Don't take a second helping just because a hostess encourages you. It is easy to rationalize and say to yourself, "I guess just this once it won't hurt. And Mary did go to so much trouble baking the lasagna because she knows how much I like it." Instead, you might try saying to yourself, "Maybe Mary likes to see me fat. Maybe it makes her feel superior having a trim body when I'm roly-poly. And I notice she isn't taking a second helping herself!" Then say out loud with a gracious smile, "No thank you, Mary. I've had plenty." There is no need to offer an excuse such as "I'm trying to lose a few pounds," or "I'm trying to stay away from too many carbohydrates." These excuses will often be countered with statements like, "Oh, you look just fine. Those extra pounds hardly show." Or, "That low-carbohydrate theory doesn't work for me at all." And you will only have to offer additional excuses. As a matter of fact, a good strategy is to leave a bite or two of food on your plate. Then you won't be offered a second helping. A bite or two of food left on the plate is not interpreted in terms of your not liking the food. It is taken by an intelligent hostess to mean that you have had enough to eat. Only an insensitive person would press additional food on you when you leave a bit of food on your plate. The food left on your plate is like a message to your hostess that says, "I enjoyed your meal. Look, I ate almost all of it. But these two or three remaining bites show that I've had quite enough and don't need or want a second helping."

You might find it helpful to make a list of the social situations in which you find it difficult to limit your intake of food. First list the social situation, and next to it place a number indicating the approximate number of times the situation occurs during the year. Here is my own list:

Birthday parties: 14
Anniversaries: 4
Dinner out with other couples: 25
Dinner at other homes: 20
Guests at our home: 25
Weddings: 4
Holidays: 8
Dinner out with colleagues: 40
Sunday picnics: 15

The grand total is 155. This means that I'm provided with about 155 social situations a year in which I might find it convenient to rationalize my eating behavior. This is the almost incredible total of one-third of the days in the year! If I were to overeat just at these times—when it is easy to kid yourself into thinking that the laws of nature have somehow been magically suspended for a moment—I would be overweight again.

Of course, the ego defense mechanism of rationalization is not restricted to social situations. It can be employed by overweight people in many ways. Have you ever heard of the "big bones" theory? A physician tells a patient, "Mrs. J., you must lose forty pounds. You have hypertension, and your heart is overtaxed by the excess poundage." On a conscious level Mrs. J. agrees with her physician. But somewhere deep inside her a little voice is whispering, "He's crazy! Can't he see you have big bones? Why if you lost forty pounds you'd be a ghost! You'd look like a living skeleton! Twenty pounds is more than enough!"

Another common rationalization is the "I have to cook for a large family" theory. A variant of this theory is an appeal to one's ethnic origins: "How can I diet? We're Italians (or Jewish, or French, etc.), doctor. And you know how Italians love to eat!"

Rationalization is a form of excuse-making for yourself. The key thing in controlling excessive rationalization is to ask yourself if the reasons you are giving for your behavior are real reasons or merely a facade—a way of kidding yourself— hiding your real motives. You must try to get behind your self-erected facade before you can understand yourself.

PROJECTION

In the ego defense mechanism called projection the subject places blame outside himself. I recall the first visit of Mary Z. She was about sixty pounds overweight, dark-haired, and neatly dressed. As she chain-smoked, she told me about her life. Her husband didn't understand her, they never discussed anything interesting or important with each other. She loved poetry and fine novels. He liked beer and the ball games on television. Most nights he was mildly "stoned" with three or four beers. He was not interested in having sexual relations with her. Sometimes months went by and he made no sexual advances. Her children were a source of great anxiety. Tommy, age 16, was stubborn and defiant. She knew he could be a straight-A student. But he just didn't try. His father wanted him to major in a profession (for example, medicine or law). But Tommy wanted to be a carpenter or an auto mechanic. He was a great disappointment. Sally, age 14, was fat just like her mother. Mrs. Z. couldn't understand this. In view of her own overweight problem, she had worked hard at making Sally aware of the dangers of overeating. She had to nag the poor child constantly to get her to eat less. And even then she sneaked food from the refrigerator and the pantry when Mrs. Z. wasn't looking. Mrs. Z. just couldn't understand Sally's willful behavior. Didn't she appreciate all that her mother was doing for her? Billy, age 8, was two years behind in his reading comprehension at school. And this was a great source of worry and anxiety.

Mrs. Z. offered this catalogue of woes as the explanation of her eating problem. She summarized her own perception of her life situation when she said, "Who wouldn't overeat with my problems? With all my worries and frustrations I have no choice. I know I turn to food the way an alcoholic turns to drink. But there's nothing I can do. I'm helpless. Unless my husband and my children change, there's nothing I can do. And they're not going to change. Especially my husband. He's hopeless."

Your first reaction when you listen to someone like Mrs. Z. is to agree with her. It does appear that all of her problems stem from the outside. Also, she states her case well. She is like a defense lawyer, abstracting from her life situation only the details relevant to support her own case. Like the defense lawyer, Mary Z. also has a client to defend—her ego. Remember, she wants to think well of herself. So it is difficult for her to place any blame on herself for her family problems. The source of her problems is *external*—everything is the fault of her husband and children. Nothing is *internal*. She refuses to see the ways in which she contributes to the family problems.

Projection is rampant in the statements of overweight persons. Here are additional examples of how overweight persons project blame outside themselves:

"My mother is my problem. She insists on taking me out to lunch three and four times a week to nice restaurants. How can you resist when you know she can afford it and wants to pay the bill?"

"My husband is a bastard. He knows how much I love malts. And he really thinks it's cute to fix rich malts in the blender for himself and the kids. Of course, he always fixes enough for me—he knows I can't resist. I know the bastard wants to see me fat. It makes him feel superior."

"It's that candy machine at work. It's in the hallway right outside my office. And I know the thing is there. Every morning when I drive to work I tell myself that I'm not going to have a candy bar today. And then I keep thinking about it. It gets to be a bigger and bigger thing in my mind until I just can't concentrate at all on what I'm doing. By ten o'clock I usually break down and have a candy bar. Then that does it. Sometimes I have three or four candy bars in a single day. Why did the good Lord let them invent candy?" (Even God is dragged into the picture, and additional blame is projected on Him.)

"It's that skinny next-door neighbor of mine, Alice. We've

been best friends ever since high school. She's always been underweight and I've always been overweight. We pick up the kids together after school. Almost every day she suggests that we stop in at one of the drive-in stands for hamburgers, tacos, or doughnuts. She knows I can't resist food, and still she does it to me. She claims she wants me to lose weight. She's my best friend, after all. But I don't think so."

"My mother is the world's best cook. Ever since I married Sally I think my mother has been trying to outdo herself to show up my wife. We go over there for dinner at least once a week, and you should see the feast my mother puts out. She always has a complete seven-course dinner. And then for dessert she usually has at least two items: cake *and* pie. Or cake *and* French pastry. What can I do? Can I insult my mother by not eating her food?"

All of these projective statements reflect a lack of insight. The blame does not lie outside oneself. The problem arises from within. The problem lies in the overweight person's reaction to a given situation. It is a question of his perceptions and attitudes toward food. No one in the world can make you eat something you really don't want. It is true that your spouse, parents, or friends may not make things easy for you. But they won't curl up and die or fly into uncontrolled rage if you suddenly reverse your habitual behavior patterns. Oh, they will be surprised. But they'll quickly get over it.

One overweight patient, David R., had a mother who always fixed large meals when he and his wife visited. (He was quoted earlier.) And he didn't know how to deal with his mother's behavior. Week after week he passively accepted the food she shoved at him. Of course, David's wife was furious with him. He tried to diet at home. He insisted on low-carbohydrate meals at home. On one of his visits he went prepared with a paperback book that described his diet. When his mother tried to offer him a piece of pie, he refused.

His mother said, "Oh, David. You know you've tried to diet before. What's the use? Have a piece of the banana pie. I cooked it just for you." This time David took out the paperback book and handed it to his mother. He said, "Mom, this is the diet I'm on. And I'm sticking to it. Don't tempt me to make exceptions. You can keep that book. It's an extra copy I bought just for you so you'll know how I want to eat from now on when I visit." His mother was somewhat taken aback. But much to David's surprise she was not angry. She could see that something was different this time, and she respected his resolve. An unexpected dividend of this little incident was that David's mother decided to lose some of her own excess poundage. David's new attitude had inspired her.

In a nutshell: nobody can make you overeat. Your weight problems are not caused by an external situation. It is your own attitudes that make you place the blame elsewhere but not on yourself—where it really belongs. The next time you are tempted to blame other people or your life situation for your overeating, ask yourself, "Am I projecting? Is this other person or situation just a convenient scapegoat for my own eating desires?"

FANTASY

One of the several ways the ego defends itself against brutal reality is by fantasy. When things get too tough for us we all have a tendency to slip into brief states of day-dreaming in which our fondest dreams are granted. Psychologists call this *autistic thinking,* and it is an outstanding characteristic of the thoughts of children. Often very young children cannot distinguish readily between their fantasy world and the real world. However, when an adult does so much autistic thinking that he cannot function in the real world, we consider him mentally ill. To a certain extent, schizophrenics in mental hospitals can be thought of as persons who have slipped out of the real world to live in a self-made world much more to their liking than the world the rest of us live in.

Although very few of us want to leave the real world completely, it is very common for us to employ fantasy as a buffer between our egos and the real world when we experience too many frustrations or conflicts. Thus the use of fantasy is normal. However, there are times when it can create blind spots even in individuals with otherwise good reality contact.

I recall one young student, Sue T. Sue was an education major. She wanted to be a teacher in the elementary grades. Her reality contact appeared to be good in all respects. She maintained a high B average in her academic subjects. She was rarely absent from class, and appeared to be a conscientious and responsible person in most respects. She was also about fifty pounds overweight. In private discussions with me she revealed a kind of dreamlike attitude about her overweight problem. She spent a lot of time daydreaming about the time when she would have her elementary school credential and become a certified teacher. In these daydreams she always saw herself as slim and beautiful. In one of her psychotherapy sessions, I asked her to close her eyes and have a controlled fantasy in which she was to describe herself five years from now. "I see myself in front of a class of first-graders. Oh, they're a nice class! See their bright, shining faces. All clean and scrubbed and neat and eager to learn. I'm putting an arithmetic problem on the board, and I see myself as if from the outside—like looking at a movie. I'm beautiful. I don't know what someone as beautiful as me is doing out here in the sticks teaching school. I should be in Hollywood or something. But it's O.K. I like to teach school. This is what I want to do. I turn around and face the children, and I see my face. It's glowing with beauty and health. My complexion—which has always been a problem—is all cleared up! Why it's amazing! My figure is fantastic—I'm a perfect size eight, and all the weight is off in just the right places."

"And how did you lose this weight?" I asked.

"Oh, I don't know. It just came off. It will. Everything is going to be all right when I get my teaching credential."

Sue had a very childish attitude toward her own very adult goal of wanting a teaching credential. Somehow the teaching credential was the "Open Sesame"—the magic key—to a whole new personality. If her hopes are shattered, if she doesn't lose weight and become a beautiful person when she begins teaching, she is bound to suffer a certain amount of frustration and depression. This is the real reason for limiting our fantasy life. Although we may achieve some or many of our goals in life, our attainments seldom match their idealized form in our fantasies.

I vividly recall Billy, a boy of twelve. He was perhaps eighty pounds overweight. He huffed and puffed just walking up and down the stairs to his classes. The other boys always chose him last when they were picking sides for a baseball team. And the only reason he was picked at all was because the teacher insisted on it. But Billy knew the other fellows really didn't want him. Knowing he wasn't wanted made him extremely tense during the games, and he was seldom able to catch or hit a ball. He wasn't brain-damaged or lacking in fundamental coordination. All psychological tests showed his perceptual-motor coordination to be completely normal. But his anxiety level was so high when he was with his peers, he wanted so badly to be accepted that he tried too hard—and of course he "goofed." If you have read *Peanuts* by Charles Schultz, you know what I'm talking about. Charlie Brown is anxious and fails often because of his very anxiety. But

Billy's problem was worse than Charlie Brown's problem.
Billy was a *fat* Charlie Brown.

Billy had taken to living almost completely in a world of
fantasy. He had discovered comic books that featured superheroes. His favorite character was Superman. He spent many
hours alone in his room or in a corner of the schoolyard
intensely poring over his comic books. He had become so
dependent upon his comic books for substitute gratification
in his life, and he identified so strongly with Superman and
the other superheroes, that he had little incentive to change
his behavior patterns. This is another example of the role that
fantasy can play in the life of the overweight person. The
fantasy life can come to dominate the psychological life of
the individual to such a point that there is little motivation to
seek gratifications in the world of reality.

You might wonder how you "break through" to a child
like Billy. It's difficult, but not impossible. In the first place,
you don't criticize him for his failings. You don't talk to him
like the proverbial Dutch uncle. He had already received
enough of this kind of treatment from well-meaning teachers
and relatives. This only reduced his self-esteem as a person
and drove him further into himself. Instead, you let the child
talk without criticizing or judging him. You let him be
himself—and you accept him as a human being. The therapist
can read and discuss Billy's comic books with him. The child
feels he can communicate with an adult that is willing to
move into his psychological world. In this particular case, the
therapist taught Billy how to play Ping-Pong. (The psychological clinic had a room for "play therapy.") By being
very friendly and encouraging, by not criticizing, the
therapist helped Billy to eventually gain confidence as a
ping-pong player. The game did not require excessive speed
on his feet, but it did require good coordination. Billy got the
message. He was not spastic after all! He was normal! It was

only a matter of time before Billy challenged another boy to a game of ping-pong in the game room at his school. You can imagine the tremendous boost it was to his ego when he won his first game! A first step had been taken in breaking through Billy's fantasy world and shaking him out of his doldrums. (It took Billy several years, but eventually he attained a normal weight.)

There's not much point in issuing instructions to you such as: "Don't fantasize." People don't obey orders so directly. If you have a great need to engage in fantasy, you will do it in spite of good intentions and well-meaning advice. However, it is possible that by knowing about fantasy as an ego defense mechanism, you may catch yourself doing it from time to time when it seems clearly inappropriate. When this occurs you can ask yourself, "Am I using fantasy as a crutch? Is it just keeping me stuck in the mud—unable to move out of my doldrums?" Asking yourself these questions can help you attain a more realistic picture of your own behavior.

REACTION FORMATION

The psychiatrist, Carl Jung, said that for any behavior trait that is overdeveloped in the conscious part of the personality, there is an opposite behavior trait buried in the unconscious part of the personality. The more well developed the conscious trait, the stronger and more deeply buried the unconscious trait. For example, Mrs. R. is very aggressive and bossy. She dominates her husband, children, and friends. Jung would say that her aggressiveness *does not* stem from feelings of intelligence and self-esteem. Quite the contrary: aggressiveness is a defense against deep feelings of inferiority. She has to compulsively keep proving her own adequacy to herself. Psychologists call this kind of pattern a *reaction formation.* The idea is that the aggressiveness has formed as a reaction against the deep feelings of inferiority. The aggressiveness is like an anti-toxin that combats the toxin of self-doubt. It keeps Mrs. R. functioning and feeling adequate as a person.

Anti-smut campaigners may in some cases be acting out a reaction formation. Mr. C. was the leader of the local decency league. He spent an inordinate amount of his time reading obscene books and seeing pornographic movies. The ostensible reason for all of this was in order to make decisions about what books and movies the decency league would approve. However, Mr. C. also suffered from ulcers, tension headaches, and various physical complaints. His physician decided these were psychosomatic in nature, and Mr. C. was referred for psychotherapy. Mr. C. was at first a very unwilling patient. He was a very proud man, and insisted that "there was nothing wrong with his head." The therapist agreed with Mr. C. Mr. C.'s difficulty was not a thought disorder, but emotional reactions that were doing damage to his body. In psychotherapy, Mr. C. gradually became aware of a number of buried psychological conflicts in his life. One of these conflicts involved his attitudes toward his wife. He had a great deal of supressed anger toward her that he was unable to express. In many ways he was much like the famous Casper Milquetoast. Everything was "Yes, dear," and "No, dear," and "May I do this for you, sweetheart?" He was unable to express honest hostility because he secretly believed he wasn't worthy of his wife. However, his covert hostility acted as a barrier in his sexual relations. He just had no desire to make sexual advances toward his wife. It was his way of punishing her for letting him be so dominated by her.

He began to develop fantasies of having affairs with other women. He was horrified by these fantasies, and felt guilty when he had them. It was against all of his religious training.

He could not even think of being unfaithful to his wife without feeling that he was a sinner. All of this culminated in his becoming the leader of the local decency league. He was tilting at windmills in order to fight his own inner desires. Psychotherapy helped him reduce the intensity of his reaction formation and transfer some of his sexual interest back where it belonged—with his wife. A reduction in internal conflict in turn brought about a reduction in psychosomatic symptoms.

Let's apply our discussion of reaction formation to the problem of weight control. Zealots in general are to be suspected of acting out reaction formations. Mrs. W. was once a compulsive eater, attaining a weight of 286 pounds when she was forty-seven years old. She was five feet, three inches in her stocking feet. She joined a local club of women who had banded together to help each other lose weight. Almost from the beginning Mrs. W. was the star of the club. In the first week she lost ten pounds. She consistently received praise and great admiration week after week for her consistent weight losses. In the incredibly short time of thirty-two weeks, she went from 286 pounds to 125 pounds! This was an average weight loss of five pounds a week! When she hit her weight loss goal of 125, shouts of success went up in the club. She was congratulated by all. The next week the club held a party in her honor, and a decorated cake was ordered from a baker. Everyone had a piece of cake but Mrs. W. Everyone was astounded by her "willpower." She continued to receive applause and congratulations.

Mrs. W. did not leave the club. She now became a member of a subgroup dedicated to keeping off weight successfully lost. Much to everyone's amazement, she continued to lose weight. She dropped from 125 to 115 to 100 to 90 pounds. She eventually weighed in at 85 pounds. But now there were no shouts of success. The other members in the club were frankly terrified. Mrs. W. looked like a refugee from a concentration camp. What was she trying to do?

She was a middle-aged woman of forty-seven, and she took to wearing mini skirts, bright lipstick, and blue eye shadow. Her weight loss had been so rapid that her formerly full face looked like a wrinkled prune. It was criss-crossed with a web of wrinkles. She looked like a corpse dressed up for her own funeral.

When she fainted at one of the club meetings, the physician-husband of one of the club members was called. After reviving Mrs. W., he insisted that she come into his office the next day. His medical interview disclosed the fact that Mrs. W. was now suffering from *anorexia*—complete loss of appetite. She had achieved her fantastic weight loss by fasting. In the beginning she had intended to fast for only the first week—to "get the diet started." But the praise and the attention of the others had been such a lift to her weak ego that she decided to fast one more week. After a few weeks of fasting, she developed a terror of food. She felt that if she took even one bite of food she would go on a compulsive eating jag and gain back all of the weight she had lost. And she was probably right. She had not changed her food attitudes or gained any self-understanding. She was still a victim of her compulsive needs.

The physician convinced Mrs. W. that she must eat or die, and slowly she began to eat a few bites of food. She completely rejected the idea of psychotherapy. She was insulted by the suggestion. For the first few days all went well—she nibbled gingerly at food—like a person testing the water before jumping in the pool. Then she jumped in! She began gorging herself. She devoured ice cream cones, candy bars, sandwiches, everything in sight. She was like a person possessed. Nothing could stop her. Her husband and children were horrified. They saw that Mrs. W. was expanding like a balloon before their very eyes. But they saw very little of the food she ate. Most of it was consumed behind their backs. Appeals to reason were of no avail. She dropped out of the weight control group, and became a semirecluse in her own home. She spent most of her time in an old bathrobe, her hair uncombed, eating candy and watching television. As of this writing, her family is trying to convince her to see a psychotherapist for her problems, but she resists all such suggestions.

Actually, the back-and-forth syndrome is a common one for overweight people. They go on a dieting jag, almost starve themselves to death in order to attain a normal weight. They lose complete control, and gain back what they lost plus additional weight. I am reminded of Mrs. C. Over a period of ten years I have seen her go from obesity to a normal weight and back again seven times. She has weighed as much as 225 and as little as 110. She has made herself into a human yo-yo. She is either compulsively dieting or compulsively eating.

It seems to me that fads or crutches of any kind in reducing only serve to reinforce potential reaction formations, and make the long-term solution to the individual's overweight problem more difficult. Oddball diets, weird exercise programs, diet pills, do not deal with root causes of the overweight person's behavior. But they do fan the flames of any zealous tendencies he may have, and they consequently often help unsettle the difficult balance the human personality must strike between its desires and what it can actually have.

The human ego must protect itself against the "slings and arrows of outrageous fortune." And so it is natural and human to employ defense mechanisms as a buffer between ourselves and the harshness of the real world. Unfortunately, this means that we have an almost infinite capacity to deceive ourselves. And we can get caught up in our own web of deception. When this happens, the ego defense mechanisms have become maladaptive. They are not helping the individual survive. They are interfering with his survival. Therefore, it behooves us to be on guard against the excessive use of ego defense mechanisms. Just knowing about them and how they work can help to some extent. Asking yourself the right question at the right time can often give you insight into your own behavior. Quiz yourself. Question your motives. Ask yourself: Am I rationalizing now? Am I projecting the blame on my spouse? Am I relying too much on the satisfaction arising from my fantasies? Is this zealous interest of mine a reaction formation? Sometimes these questions can prick the bubble of our ego defenses, and we can see ourselves in a clearer light. When this occurs, an important first step has been taken in the direction of behavior change.

Chapter 4

Overeating Is a Habit

If there is one thing that psychologists understand, it is the psychology of hunger in animals. Hungry dogs have been taught to drool for meat powder at the sound of a bell. Hungry rats have been taught to press bars and run mazes for chow pellets. Hungry pigeons have been taught to peck at lighted discs for grain. And monkeys have been taught to rake in bananas and oranges located outside of their cages. Some critics of animal experiments have pointed out that for years they were almost exclusively concerned with hunger as a motive. It was only recently that animal experiments began to deal with other motives such as sex and curiosity.

I don't want to mislead you. Most of these experiments were not concerned with the problem of overeating behavior.

They were concerned with the acquisition and the breaking of habits in general—not just eating habits. Nevertheless, they shed quite a bit of light on human behavior when overeating is regarded as a habit. These experiments give us some idea of why our own behavior is difficult to control. They also point the way to possible strategies of self-control. Information gleaned from these experiments has been utilized in an approach to psychotherapy called *behavior modification*. The behavior modification approach makes the eating habits themselves the target of attack. Although a few behavior modification therapists may acknowledge somewhat grudgingly the role of unconscious motives in common overeating problems, they stress the fact that the overeating behavior itself is above all a habit—a fixed or stereotyped way of responding. That is why self-understanding and insight are not enough. After a person achieves some degree of insight, he still needs to change his fixed habits. Some behavior modification therapists would argue that it is well to start on habit-breaking routines even before insight is achieved. It is argued that insight and self-understanding often follow somewhat automatically as eating habits improve. This makes sense. As people lose weight their self-esteem rises. As their self-esteem rises, their egos gather strength. As their egos gather strength, they need to do less repressing of unpleasant thoughts—they can take a stiffer dose of reality about themselves. And thus many previously repressed ideas and motives tend to become spontaneously conscious.

It isn't necessary to be a purist about this. Your goal is not to resolve academic disputes between theories of unconscious motivation and behavior modification. A two-pronged approach is best. While you work at understanding your motives and ego defense mechanisms, you can also work at breaking old habits. The two approaches are compatible.

YOU ARE CONDITIONED

If you go to motion pictures, you have heard about the mysterious Russians and their "conditioning" techniques. These conditioning techniques are presented as mysterious methods of "brainwashing" prisoners of war and controlling minds. Books such as *1984* by George Orwell portray the possibility of a horrible future for mankind in which Pavlovian techniques are used to bend minds into submission with a dictatorial government. All of this sounds mysterious and occult to the uninitiated. But in fact Pavlov's techniques are far from mysterious and occult. They are straightforward methods of establishing and breaking habits that are taught in every university in the United States.

Ivan Pavlov was a great Russian physiologist who won a Nobel Prize for his studies of the digestive glands. One of the things he noticed was that his experimental animals (dogs) salivated in anticipation of being fed. When they heard the footsteps of their regular feeder in the hall, they would salivate even before the food arrived. Not only that, they could tell the footsteps of a regular feeder from the footsteps of a stranger walking down the hall. Pavlov called this act of salivating to the footsteps a "psychic secretion"—the implication being that dogs are obviously not born with the behavioral pattern of salivating to footsteps in the hall. They are born with the behavioral pattern of salivating to food in the mouth. Thus the act of anticipation represented by salivating to footsteps in the hall had to be a learned phenomenon—a habit. Pavlov wanted to study this habit in greater detail, and he devised ways of doing it.

In order to have a more readily controllable stimulus than footsteps in the hall, he decided to place experimental animals in a restraining harness in a laboratory under controlled conditions. He rang a bell just a moment before squirting meat powder into the animal's mouth. After a number of trials in which the bell and meat powder were closely paired in time, he gave the dog a test trial. "Lo and behold" the dog salivated to the bell alone! A "psychic secretion" had been created by experiment. Further pairings of the bell and meat powder were administered to the dog. And test trials subsequently revealed that the dog issued copious amounts of saliva when it heard the bell. It was almost as if the dog was confusing the bell with food. It might be better to simply say that the bell made the dog anticipate getting fed, and the saliva given to the bell was in preparation for food in the mouth. Be that as it may, a new reaction existed with a number of interesting implications. One interesting implication is the obviously *involuntary* aspect of the conditioning technique. A conditioned dog is helpless to inhibit its salivation when the bell rings. The conditioning is of the autonomic nervous system, not of the somatic nervous system. And self-control is not feasible under these circumstances for a dog. The bell rings and he salivates. That's all there is to it. Let's remember this interesting and important fact for future reference.

In the jargon of conditioning theory, the bell is a *conditioned stimulus.* That is to say, it is a previously neutral stimulus now capable of evoking a conditioned or learned reaction. Conditioned stimuli could be broadly defined as any stimuli that trigger habits. Once an animal is conditioned can it ever be deconditioned? The answer is yes, and the deconditioning technique is fairly obvious. Just present the bell a number of times without food. At first the dog will drool in large amounts at the sound of the bell. But in time he will unlearn his salivation habit, and the sound of the bell will no longer trigger the involuntary salivation. This procedure is called *extinction*—and it is the best and most reliable of all habit-breaking methods. Deconditioning cannot be accomplished all at once. If a deconditioned dog is tested after several days of rest, he will give some saliva at the sound of a bell. This is called *spontaneous recovery*—the seemingly erased habit has come back unbidden and without training. However, if the extinction procedure is gone through again, the habit can in time be completely erased for all practical purposes.

What does all of this have to do with you? Let me tell a story related to me recently by a friend. Here's the story in his own words. "I work as a tailor in a clothing factory in downtown Los Angeles. At 9:30 A.M. the bell rings for a fifteen minute coffee break, and everybody makes a mad dash for the coffee catering cart on the bottom floor. I've been making the same mad dash with everybody else for years. But now I'm trying to lose weight, and so I remain at my sewing machine. But my stomach seems to be churning with hunger. When the other fellows come back with Danish rolls and coffee I'm almost not able to stand it. I can't figure it out. I had a good breakfast at 7:30 A.M. at home, and I shouldn't be that hungry. But I am. What do you make of it? Is it psychological? Is it all in my mind?"

The story made me laugh because I was planning to write this chapter at the time I heard it, and immediately realized just how appropriate it was. It was almost too perfect to be true. But I assure you that the story was actually related to me as I told it to you. I was amazed at how well it fit the Pavlovian concept. The 9:30 bell operates for my friend in exactly the same manner as the bell in the Pavlovian experiment. It is a conditioned stimulus, and it triggers the involuntary action of the autonomic nervous system. My friend was making the same mad dash with his friends for years, and so he was well conditioned. Bell and food have been paired many times. The hunger pangs are uncontrollable. No amount of willpower in the world can make them go away. They are real. What's the answer? How can he get over this problem?

The answer is identical to the one given in the dog experiment. Deconditioning can only take place if the conditioned stimulus is presented a number of times without food. In other words he must hear the 9:30 bell, and see his friends eating Danish rolls without eating, himself. The first week will be the worst. After that it will get easier and easier. In time he will find that the bell and the sight of food don't produce the involuntary contractions of the stomach. There are other things he can do to ease the deconditioning process. For example, he can get up and leave the room while his friends are eating. But little or no actual deconditioning will take place when he does this. This is useful only if a person feels that he is going to break down and eat something. If one's conscious desire to lose weight is high at a given moment, it is far better to remain in the presence of the conditioned stimuli than to escape from them. Deconditioning takes place in their presence—not in their absence.

Let me give you an example from my own experience. I put on water to boil for instant Sanka at about 11:00 P.M. most evenings. For years I felt I had to have a snack with the Sanka. The hot Sanka and food were paired many times in my experience. The hot Sanka had become a conditioned stimulus that triggered involuntary hunger pangs. I thought I just had to have something to eat with the Sanka. It looked impossible to resist. I had let myself creep up to 196 pounds from a previous low of 173 pounds, and I knew I had to do something about it. I also knew that the late evening snack was unnecessary. I had eaten an adequate dinner, and the extra carbohydrates in cookies, ice cream, cake, or pie were really quite unnecessary. At first I tried just removing the conditioned stimulus (the Sanka) for a few weeks. But I missed the warm Sanka and its relaxing effect in the late evening. But when I began to have it again, I found I was hungry again. No deconditioning had taken place. I decided to ride it out the hard way. Every evening I had Sanka, and I said to myself, "Okay, you're hungry and you want food. You can't help the hunger contractions. They're involuntary. But you're not one of Pavlov's dogs. You're a human being, and you can ride it out." Overriding the hunger pangs in this way was difficult for the first week or so. After that the involuntary hunger came on with less and less strength. Now I can enjoy my hot cup of Sanka at night without feeling deprived or sorry for myself. The connection between the Sanka and the food has been broken.

As I write this, I realize that long ago I broke the morning coffee-break habit of having a doughnut or pastry with coffee. For years I have had nothing to eat with my friends when we take our morning coffee break. And I can honestly say that I do not feel deprived or hungry. It was so long ago that I broke the habit (circa 1952) that it doesn't even occur to me to return to having a snack in the morning. Such is the power of habits that the good habit becomes more or less unconscious too! This is the hopeful or upbeat side of the conditioning coin.

We must realize that we are conditioned in many and in subtle ways. The clock itself presents conditioned stimuli. Just seeing the hands point at 10:00, 12:00, 3:00, etc. triggers conditioned responses. Many people feel they just have to have lunch at 12:00. The noon whistle blows (another conditioned stimulus), and they feel an almost un-bearable hunger. This hunger is involuntary, and is triggered by the sight of the clock, the sound of a bell or whistle, and the sight of other people eating. It pays just to know that these are conditioned stimuli and that the principles of condi-tioning operate in us. Only then can we begin to achieve a certain freedom from conditioned stimuli. A dog cannot say to himself, "This is a conditioned stimulus. I will decondition if I expose myself to it without reward for a period of time." Thus a dog can be deconditioned only if he is manipulated by a human trainer. That is why the principles of habit-breaking for human beings are different than for dogs. A human being is more flexible in his behavior, and he can take advantage of his human insights in his attempt to break undesirable habits. A human being in a sense rises above himself and is capable of acting as his own trainer.

Food associations of all kinds are further examples of Pavlovian conditioning. People say, "I can't stand coffee without sugar," or "I have to have french fries when I have a hamburger," or "I can't stand to eat my food without bread." In each of these cases the connection between one food item and the other food item is a form of conditioning. A person tastes black coffee after years of drinking it with cream and sugar, wrinkles up his mouth, and assumes that he just doesn't like black coffee. It doesn't occur to him that his reaction is not inborn, that instead it is learned. The need for sugar or sweetening in your coffee is in the majority of cases simply a conditioned reaction that can be extinguished by drinking black coffee for a week or two. It is important to understand that the desire for sugar is a conditioned response and that it will extinguish in a brief time. If you do not know this, if you assume the preference is fixed in your constitution, then you obviously don't feel you can do anything about it. You assume that there is no habit to be worked with, and consequently you continue to feel that you absolutely must sweeten your coffee. I assure you that in the vast majority of cases it is a habit, and it can be broken. A number of people I know have given up sugar with coffee, and now they prefer black coffee. They have developed a new habitual preference such that they wrinkle up their faces when they try sugar in coffee—it tastes "too sweet."

Mr. G. was used to eating bread with all of his meals. He ate three slices of buttered toast with ham and eggs for breakfast. For lunch he had two rolls with his meat and vegetables. With dinner he had four slices of bread. When his physician suggested that he try eating some meals entirely without bread, he declared, "That's impossible for me. I have to have bread with my meals. I gag on plain steak and vegetables. They just don't go down." Mr. G. had been raised in a family that simply assumed you always have bread with every meal. This was a habit well established since childhood. Mr. G.'s physician assured him that he might have a hard time eating a meal without bread at first, but that if he tried it a few times he would find it quite possible to do. The first goal was to cut out bread with his dinner. After two weeks he reported to his physician that it had not been nearly as difficult as he thought it would be. Here is his own report: "The first evening meal without bread was really bad. I thought that you were crazy. I would never learn to eat a meal without bread. After all, I had eaten bread with every meal all my life since I don't know when. But I tried it. My wife had fixed a broiled steak, asparagus, and a tossed green salad. I ate the meal with no pleasure at all. I felt completely deprived. But I must admit that my gagging theory was all off. I had no trouble swallowing. I just felt sorry for myself. Why did I have to suffer this way? The next night was a little better, and the next night was even easier. By the end of the week I almost had reached the point where I didn't miss bread with my meals. Now I don't miss it at all. As a matter of fact—I know you won't believe this—I think I prefer my dinner without bread. I can taste the food better. Before I was stuffing big bites of bread into my mouth with all of the other food, and I had my mouth so loaded that I couldn't taste a thing. I look back on that way of eating and it disgusts me. This is simply amazing to me. I never realized that eating bread with my meals was just a habit—and a habit that wasn't particularly hard to break."

Although we are creatures of habit, there is nothing absolute or completely fixed about habits. Habits are not poured in concrete. They exist in your nervous system. And your nervous system is alive and flexible. Long-standing habits are sometimes not as difficult to change as people think they are.

A DIFFERENT KIND OF CONDITIONING

So far we have been speaking of only one kind of conditioning, Pavlovian conditioning. The habits acquired on the basis of Pavlovian conditioning involve the autonomic nervous system, and do not fall within the domain of what we usually call freely willed behavior. (For example, my tailor friend's stomach contractions were involuntary when the 10:00 A.M. break arrived.) However, there is another kind of conditioning—*instrumental conditioning*—which involves the conditioning of the somatic nervous system. And this does fall into the classification of what we normally think of as voluntary behavior or behavior that is under the control of our will. B. F. Skinner, Harvard research psychologist, has studied this behavior in great detail, and shown how it is much more under the control of the *reinforcement principle* than it is under the control of a hypothetical will.

Before we discuss human applications let us review Skinner's basic experiments with rats. A rat is placed in an instrumental conditioning apparatus (popularly called a "Skinner box"). The apparatus has a bar that can be easily depressed by the animal, and a food cup. Whenever the animal depresses the bar, a pellet of food falls into the cup. At first an animal placed in a Skinner box just wanders around—explores. He sniffs here and there in an apparently random pattern. Even if he is hungry, he does not press the bar. In time he will inadvertently depress the bar. The food pellet falls in the cup, and the hungry rat eats it. Now if the rat had high intelligence or what we call human insight, he would look at the bar and the food and say to himself, "Hey, pretty good deal! When I press the bar I get food." He would make the connection swiftly, and soon he would be merrily bar pressing for food pellets. But the rat does not make a quick connection. He eats the pellet but apparently does not see that his own act of bar pressing brought the pellet. However, through a process of trial and error he finally becomes an avid bar presser. A rat that has been in the Skinner box for a few hours is bar pressing at a high rate for food. In the terminology of instrumental conditioning, food is the *reinforcer* for the act of bar pressing. This form of learning is called *instrumental conditioning* because the act of bar pressing is instrumental in bringing food or reinforcement to the animal.

Now let's pretend that bar pressing is a bad habit. We want the animal to get rid of it. How would you do it? Would you say to the animal, "Hey, you in there. Stop pressing the bar. That's just a dirty, nasty habit and I want you to give it up." The rat might be attracted by the sound of your voice and look at you a moment. But he would quickly return to his bar-pressing behavior. He can't understand English in the first place, and in the second place he "knows" that his habit brings him something he wants no matter what you say. (The example, while facetious, is meant to apply to parents who try to use simple admonition to get their children to give up habits that are obviously reinforcing to the child.) Maybe you could punish the rat. Every time he presses the bar slap his paws. This has been tried. A little apparatus has been attached to the bar, and this apparatus comes down and slaps the rat's paw every time he presses the bar. The effects of such punishment are not permanent. After a substantial amount of punishment the habit persists. When the punishment is removed, the rat goes back to bar pressing at his old high rate. Nothing has been accomplished. The habit is still there, and the animal has suffered.

No, the only reliable way to extinguish the animal is to withhold reinforcement—the food pellets. Gradually, the rat will give up his bar-pressing habit if he sees it doesn't pay off. He'll keep working at it for quite a while, but his rate of bar pressing will inevitably come down and eventually fall almost to zero if we stop feeding him when he presses the bar. And it's that simple. A strong habit is erased by nonreinforcement.

In my psychology classes students often object to the Skinner experiment. A student may say, "Is the implication that this is how men behave? Man is not a rat. The rat acts like a robot. A man has will, intelligence, reasoning, logic, religion, and creativity. The principles of human behavior are not the same as rat behavior."

My answer to that is, "Yes, all that you say is true. However, we can learn something from the rats. There are certain similarities in their behavior and in our behavior. As a matter of fact, one way we rise above simple rat behavior is by understanding the principles of instrumental conditioning. Then we can do something about them when we see them operating in ourselves. This, of course, the rat cannot do."

All right. What are the human implications? It seems to me that the biggest implication of the reinforcement principle is that behavior is shaped by its own consequences. You execute an action. If it pays off, the likelihood of executing that action again goes up. If it does not pay off, the likelihood of executing that action goes down. Well-established habits are behaviors that have frequently paid off for us in the past. We engage in them because they bring us reinforcement. This is where our previous discussion of unconscious motivation enters the picture. Your overeating habit may be getting you something you were not aware of. As previously explained, overeating may be a way of reducing anxiety, expressing aggression, avoiding sexual relations, avoiding people, etc. These are all the "payoffs" or reinforcers for the act of overeating. You're getting what you want out of overeating. That's why lectures, exhortations, and the usual good advice are all worthless. They don't cut to the roots of the problem. The key to extinction, then, is the withholding of reinforcement when this is at all feasible.

Let's take an actual illustration of how this has been done in psychotherapy with human beings, and then we'll try to make applications to you. Two research psychologists, Halmuth Schaefer and Patrick Martin, at Patton State Hospital in California, decided to do something about over-weight mental patients. Remember, the patients were locked up, and so the statements made about their treatment only have partial implications for the treatment of persons who are free to put themselves into and out of certain eating situations. Nevertheless, their research is important and we can learn from it.

A nurse sits at a table with an overweight patient, Miss Y. The nurse speaks to the patient only when the patient is not eating. The patient is encouraged to speak a complete sentence between every mouthful of food. It thus takes "forever" to eat. The nurse praises the patient if the patient leaves food on the dish or dawdles over the food. Notice that the nurse's behavior is almost the mirror opposite of what the average parent does in a typical child-rearing situation.

Children are encouraged to finish all their food, not take "forever" to eat, etc. No wonder that there are so many overweight children, and—as a consequence—so many overweight adults. The habits established in childhood carry over into adult life. The method of Schaefer and Martin gives reinforcement (i.e., attention, praise) to any actions associated with eating less, eating more slowly, leaving food, etc. It also gives nonreinforcement to any action of eating (e.g., the patient is ignored when she is eating). It is not surprising that they had excellent results with their patients. The method of treatment was direct, effective, and relatively painless for the patient.

The same method can be applied to eating between meals. Let us say that a patient has had a habit of eating a candy bar in the afternoon. The nurse need not criticize her when she sees her eating a candy bar. This is ignored. Criticism would act like punishment, and only temporarily suppress the habit. The patient will probably try to find a way to eat the candy bar behind the nurse's back. Instead, the nurse can attempt to shape the extinction of the candy-bar habit gradually. Let us say that the patient usually buys the candy at 3:00 P.M. One day the nurse notes that the candy bar is not purchased until 4:00 P.M. The nurse can day, "I see you waited until 4:00 o'clock to have your candy bar." One day the patient does not buy a candy bar. The nurse should encourage this action by saying, "I see you were able to skip the candy bar today. That's great!" What the nurse is doing is simply this: she is reinforcing the act of not eating, and she is ignoring the act of eating.

Of course, this procedure may backfire. Some patients are so hostile that they do not respond to praise. If the relationship between the nurse and the patient is a poor one, praise may do more harm than good. In this case praise simply cannot be used. It is, in fact, not a reinforcer. It only superficially looks like a reinforcer. A reinforcer is defined as any stimulus that increases the probability of a response. And if praise does not increase the probability of a response for a particular patient, then it is not a reinforcer. A suitable reinforcer must be found. A helpful guide for finding suitable reinforcers to control behavior has been suggested by David Premack of the University of California at Santa Barbara. This is discussed in the next section.

PREMACK'S PRINCIPLE

David Premack has suggested a practical way of figuring out what will and what will not act as a reinforcer. The principle makes a great deal of sense, and can be described in a general way as follows:

1. Select any two behavioral acts of an organism for study.
2. Rank the acts according to their probability of occurrence. Let's call the act with the lowest probability Act 1. The act with the highest probability is Act 2.
3. Arrange matters in such a way that the low-probability act (Act 1) must be performed by the organism in order to attain the opportunity to engage in the high-probability act (Act 2).
4. The probability of Act 1 will go up, and the probability of Act 2 will go down.
5. Act 2 is a reinforcer for Act 1.

Practical applications of the principle in the field of mental health abound. Here is Johnny, age 8, an autistic child. He is an obscure patient on a ward for the mentally retarded. But he is not mentally retarded in the usual sense of the word. His apparent lack of intelligence is partly due to his complete withdrawal from reality. He has a favorite chair, and he sits and rocks on this chair for hours each day. You go into the ward and see him sitting like a little ball on the chair rocking hour after hour in a stereotyped rhythm. It is a pathetic sight. What can be done? The application of Premack's principle can be an important step in helping the child attain reality contact. Let's say that Johnny should go outside and get some sunshine and fresh air for at least a portion of the day. He is very reluctant to do this. But his therapist thinks he should. Rocking in the chair is obviously a high-probability act. Going outside to play is obviously a low-probability act. We must arrange matters in such a way that Johnny cannot rock on the chair unless he goes outside for a certain period of time. This may be easier said than done. But if the therapist and the others who work with Johnny persist, they will be well rewarded for their efforts. In time Johnny will willingly go outside in order to get to his favorite activity: chair rocking. But, interestingly, the amount of chair rocking will also tend to decrease. The systematic application of Premack's principle to a variety of behavioral acts can go a long way in breaking through Johnny's shell of withdrawal.

Let's try an application of Premack's principle to a weight control problem. Jane Q. is an overweight mental patient. She weighs over 300 pounds, and takes second and third helpings at the dining table. We can define *eating less* at the dining room table as a low-probability response. We also note that Jane is very talkative. She eats with her mouth full and tends to dominate the conversation at a table she shares with other patients. Jane claims she wants to lose weight, and will cooperate with the suggestions of the therapist. Jane is highly intelligent and can comprehend Premack's principle when it is explained to her. The therapist suggests that she make a little internal promise to herself: she will not say anything at the table until she decides that she is completely done eating. Until the discussion of Premack's principle, Jane was not fully aware of her own behavior. Eating and talking were all mixed up for her into one big activity. Now the activities were made distinct for her by the discussion with the therapist. We find that she begins eating somewhat less in order to get to talk. And we also find that talking at the table decreases—a joy to the other patients.

A friend of mine, a heavy smoker, recently asked me how he could cut down on his smoking. I noticed that he smoked as he talked. So I suggested that he simply decide that he would never talk and smoke at the same time. When chatting with friends he was to promise himself that if he lit up a cigarette he would cease talking until he put out the cigarette. Putting out the cigarette (low-probability behavior) was made the instrumental act for attaining the freedom to talk (high-probability behavior). He is finding that thinking this way about his own behavior is making it possible for him to reduce his smoking in social situations. He smokes fewer cigarettes, and he often smokes only a small part of a cigarette. Smoking silently he becomes impatient with the smoking, wants to talk, and willingly puts out the cigarette.

You can apply Premack's principle to yourself. It involves two things: (1) analyzing your own behavior patterns, and (2) making an internal agreement with yourself. Let us say that you are a homemaker and you have developed a habit of having a dish of ice cream as a part of your lunch. You want to cut out the ice cream (low-probability). Right after lunch you watch your favorite television serial (high-probability). Promise yourself that if you do not have the ice cream, you may watch the serial. This is the only "willpower" you have to use. Don't try to use your willpower to say, "I'm not going to have the ice cream." Go ahead and have the ice cream if you want it badly, but don't watch the television serial if you do. If you really give this an honest try, you will find that you *want* to give up the ice cream.

Of course, this may not work for you if the probability of eating the ice cream is even greater than the probability of watching the television serial. If this is the case, you may have to cast about for some other behavior of yours that is even more probable than eating the ice cream. Perhaps you enjoy reading. You have just purchased a novel you want to get into. Promise yourself you won't read any of the novel for one day if you have the ice cream with your lunch. These are only examples, of course. Only you know and understand your own behavior patterns.

One of my patients, Miss G., was an aspiring author. She was a single schoolteacher, lived alone, and was working on a novel that she planned to submit to a New York publisher. She walked home from work and passed a bakery on the way home. This bakery had become Temptation incarnate for her. Every day when leaving work she vowed that she would not stop in and buy anything. And almost every day she lost her self-control and bought some kind of baked item. She wanted to know what she could do about the situation. It would have been possible to simply avoid the bakery entirely. This would have meant several extra blocks of walking. And the exercise would have done her good. However, she wanted to be able to walk right by the bakery and not buy anything. There were two reasons for this: (1) There was the matter of self-esteem. She wanted to be able to say to herself that she had "licked" this thing. (2) No real deconditioning would take place if she avoided the bakery. Remember, deconditioning takes place only in the *presence* of the conditioned stimuli. If she could learn to decondition herself to the bakery, this deconditioning might spread to baked goods in general. Thus, she would not only be able to pass the bakery, but there would also be the additional benefit that she could start to pass up baked goods during social occasions.

I suggested that she try Premack's principle as a booster to her strong conscious desire to pass up the bakery. It was her practice to arrive home about 4:30 P.M. and work on her novel for two hours. She ate a late dinner—about 7:30 P.M., and if she had no social engagement, spent the evening reading a novel or books on the art of writing. She seldom failed to put in two hours working on her novel—obviously a very high probability behavior. If she bought baked goods, she was not to do any work on the novel. If she passed up the baked goods, she could "reward" herself by working on the novel.

The first two days she failed to pass by the bakery. And she kept the promise to herself of not writing. But by the third day she was so frustrated at not being able to work on the novel, that when she left work she knew she would be able to pass by the bakery and not buy anything. Let's hear it from her in her own words:

"By the third day of trying Premack's principle, I was just bursting with unexpressed ideas for the novel. When I left work I was actually looking forward to walking right by the bakery! I walked briskly in the direction of the bakery, and I almost stuck my tongue out at it. I walked right by, and deliberately slowed down so that I could look in the window and tempt myself. But no problem. I just kept on walking. What a thrill! You have no idea what a kick it was that first day I walked by that bakery."

Here is a later report, after two weeks: "Still no problem. One day I almost went in. But I just thought to myself, 'Okay, you can go in if you want to. But if you do, remember you can't work on the novel this afternoon.' This thought just about completely demolished my desire to enter the bakery. I was filled with images of what I was going to write that afternoon. And the thought of not writing was almost intolerable to me. When you first proposed Premack's principle I thought it was sort of silly—just a game. But it has helped me to analyze my own behavior, and I can verify that it is working for me. Also, it's true that I'm not as tempted by cookies, pies, cake, etc. when I'm invited out. You spoke of a 'generalization' of the deconditioning effect, and this seems to be working out."

Of course, no single principle is the whole answer to a weight problem. Premack's principle is, however, a helpful aid to weight control. Give it a try. You will find it helpful in analyzing your actual behavior patterns, and in getting a clearer insight into what is and what is not important to you.

MOTIVATION AND REINFORCEMENT

You will recall that earlier in this chapter I suggested that the biggest implication of Skinner's work is that behavior is shaped by its own consequences. I said that your overeating habit may be getting you something of which you are not completely aware. The purpose of these comments is to build a bridge between the basic concepts of Freud and the basic concepts of Skinner. Freud believed that unconscious motives are very important in human behavior. Thus the overweight person, as already indicated, may overeat to express aggression in a passive manner, avoid sexual relations, etc. To the extent that these motives are repressed or denied to the self, to that extent is the problem compounded. Skinner does not speak of unconscious motives. Instead, he speaks of the reinforcement principle. In order to extinguish an unwanted behavior it is necessary to withhold reinforcement. Although Skinner does not see eye to eye with Freud on a number of theoretical issues, it is clear that both men are expressing in somewhat different terms the great importance of motivational concepts. To me, the goal of an unconscious motive can be conceptualized as the "target" or "payoff" or "reinforcer" for a behavioral act. If the goal of a particular overweight person is to be offensive to a spouse by being overweight, and if the spouse gets "uptight" over the partner's weight problem, then getting uptight acts as a reinforcer to perpetuate the weight problem. If the over- weight partner is unaware of his or her motivation, there is little hope for changing behavior. That is why the first step is to analyze your own motives as suggested in Chapter 2. This is the way you "break through" and discover what is rein- forcing your overeating habit. Once you see the target of a motive—the reinforcer—you can ask yourself other questions: What can I do about this? Is there any other way I can gain the same satisfaction by other means?

One patient, Mrs. R., could never tell her husband that she was angry. When he criticized her, she pouted and ate behind his back. He was very critical of her housekeeping, and she never defended herself. She felt the criticism was unjustified, of course. And the more he criticized her, the worse her housekeeping became. He also hated her fatness. And the more he hated her fatness, the fatter she became. In psycho- therapy, she became quickly aware of the passive-aggressive aspects of her overeating. She saw that it was a way of punishing her husband for treating her like a child. She also became aware of why she couldn't speak her mind to him. Her own mother had often slapped Mrs. R's face when she "sassed" her back. She had developed a behavior pattern of pouting and sneaking food as a child. This carried over into adult life, and she was unconsciously expecting her husband to slap her if she "sassed" him back. She was encouraged to express her aggression openly instead of hiding it within herself. She finally got up her courage. And one day when he made some comments about the furniture being dusty, she told him, "What do you expect on a hot day when I have to keep the windows open? We don't have air conditioning, and a house with open windows just gets dusty. Let's install a central air-conditioning unit if you can't stand a little dust!"

Mrs. R. reported that she could feel a certain terror of anticipation as she spoke. She expected a heavy hand to crash against her face. But much to her surprise, her husband took it fairly well. They had a few cross words. But he certainly didn't hit her. Her comments opened up a discussion about the feasability of installing air conditioning, and in a few weeks she happily reported that her husband had agreed to the installation of a central unit. As her anger toward her husband diminished, she had less need for food—less need to hurt him. The real motive for much of her eating behavior was unexpressed aggression towards her husband. One of the "reinforcers" or "payoffs" for her behavior was the pained expression on her husband's face when she took another piece of pie or waddled into the room. As she found better ways to express aggression, she had less need to see his pained expression—less need to hurt him. As a consequence, she was able to change her eating patterns.

You can see that although the language chosen by Freud and Skinner to talk about behavior is different, there are certain essential similarities in their approaches. If you are to lose weight, you must simultaneously become aware of your unconscious motives and become aware of the target of these motives—the reinforcers or "payoffs" that keep your overeating behavioral patterns going. You overeat for reasons. What are the payoffs?

The principles discussed in this chapter are sound. They work. But let's admit that they are difficult to apply to ourselves. It is one thing for a parent to apply them to the rearing of a child, or for a psychotherapist to apply them to a patient. It is quite another thing to be both the subject and the object of the application of a conditioning principle. In order to do this you have to almost "go outside" of your own skin. You have to visualize yourself as another person would see you. You must, in essence, become objective about your own behavior. It is difficult, but it can be done. This is the great advantage human beings have over animals. Although many human beings obviously cannot be objective about their own behavior, many human beings can. They can stand back a moment from themselves, analyze their behavior, and make changes. It is language that gives us the ability to do this. A human being can express in words the principles of conditioning, something an animal cannot do. Thus an animal is completely bound by the principles of conditioning. But a man can reflect, verbalize a principle, and no longer be its prisoner. By the same token, you can verbalize a principle such as Premack's principle and apply it to yourself. Again, this is not easy to do—but neither is it impossible. We must not confuse difficulty with nonfeasability. Human beings can work at breaking their own bad habits and can succeed in their goal. I cannot by any stretch of the imagination conceive of any animal doing this. A dog, rat, or pigeon cannot say to itself, "Oh, I see. In this situation I am responding to the hamburger the same way Pavlov's dog responds to the bell. The hamburger has become a conditioned stimulus that triggers my desire for French fries." And not being able to say this kind of thing to itself, a dog, rat, or pigeon cannot by an act of intention break a habit. Human consciousness makes it possible for you to break bad habits.

Chapter 5

Psychological Exercises

In order to break bad habits, it is helpful to become more aware of the details of the behavior involved in the execution of the bad habit. This principle was first formulated by the psychologist Knight Dunlap with his justly famous principle of *negative practice*. Negative practice simply means that you consciously and deliberately practice your bad habit. As an illustration, let us say that you make a particular typing error. You type "ht" every time you want to type "th." This is obviously quite a nuisance. What can you do to break the habit? Dunlap suggested that you sit at the typewriter and consciously and deliberately type the error—"ht"—over and over again. You might do this ten minutes at a time, three times a day for one week. You will find that it is almost impossible to make the error when you are doing regular typing work. In the past you made the error more or less unconsciously—the habit operated out of the center of your consciousness and was not under your voluntary control. But by practicing the error you have become so aware of the bad habit that it is almost impossible to make it.

Before we attempt to apply the principle of negative practice to the specific problem of overeating, let us give another illustration of an application of the principle. Joseph Sheean of the U.C.L.A. psychology department, is one of the foremost speech therapists in the United States. His method of treating persons with a stuttering problem utilizes to a large degree the principle of negative practice. The stutterer is encouraged to stutter consciously and deliberately even at times when he would not have a tendency to stutter. Sheean's clients are given exercises in which they must engage strangers in conversation and then intentionally stutter. For example, the assignment might be to stop a stranger and ask the time of day. Even if the stutterer has an "attack of fluency" he is to *pretend* that he stutters. By thus consciously practicing his undesirable behavior he begins to bring it under conscious control.

Now let's apply the principle of negative practice to the problem of overeating. The application of the principle involves designing psychological exercises which make it possible for the overweight person to become more conscious of (1) what he actually does on a behavioral level when he overeats, and (2) his thoughts and feelings when he overeats. In order to accomplish these dual goals, exercises were designed which require the overweight person to respond to food in atypical ways. Overeating is a complex problem involving both unconscious motivation and stereotyped ways of responding to foods (i.e., habits). The purpose of the exercises which are described in the following pages is to put some "static" between the stimulus (food) and the habitual response to it (eating). This helps to "short-circuit" the habit.

EATING IN FRONT OF A MIRROR

The first exercise is simply called "eating in front of a mirror." The name of the exercise is self-explanatory. These are the instructions:

Do this exercise only when you are alone and have complete privacy. You do not need anyone's approval or disapproval for *any* of the exercises described in this book.

If you have a portable mirror, bring it to the kitchen table. If you do not have a portable mirror, go into a bedroom or bathroom with some favorite food. Now just eat the food in front of the mirror in as normal a fashion as possible.

Watch yourself closely. Try to observe as many details of your behavior as possible. Do you eat with your mouth open or closed? Do you take big or small bites? How do your cheeks look as you eat? What thoughts are going through your head as you do this exercise? Take notes on your reactions *at the moment* they occur to you. It is all right to interrupt the exercise to jot down notes. Don't wait until after the exercise, or you will forget to get down some important points.

Here are the reactions of several clients to the exercise:

"By eating in front of a mirror it made me self-conscious of my double chin, how I chew my food, and how my complexion was getting along. By watching myself it made me sick to watch and I stopped eating."

"Eating in front of the mirror proved to be a very uncomfortable experience. I eat so fast and watching myself literally shoveling it in was really gross. I found myself taking smaller bites simply because I never realized that my cheeks were so enormous. Seeing myself as others see me is really something! If I had to eat in front of a mirror all the time I'm sure I'd be eating more carrot sticks than peanut butter sandwiches."

"By watching myself eat I could see how it looks when I 'gobble' food. After doing it several times, I found myself eating much slower, therefore, getting fuller faster."

"Last week when I ate in front of a mirror it made me angry—with myself, but it was a frustrating anger. When I did the exercise this past week, I felt disgust with myself. I couldn't pinpoint why I felt disgust. Was (or rather *is*) it the act of eating, loss of self-esteem, or am I angry at the food going into my mouth? I don't like this exercise but the fact that it bothers me so, I am determined to face it when I get the nerve to take the reaction I undergo. I only do this once a week because I can't imagine seeing myself more often—I 'see' myself enough from that 'slap in the face' once a week."

"First of all, watching anyone eat is not exactly my favorite thing. Somehow the chewing, sloshing, chomping action is ridiculous to see. Upon viewing myself in this action I am reminded of 'Bossie the Cow' chewing her cud in the pasture. Embarrassment, disgust and a sense of the ridiculous are my initial feelings. However, as I continued I evolved into self-hate, and mountains of self-pity. In a word, what I see is: Sickening. . . ."

As you can see from the reactions, eating in front of a mirror can be a powerful technique for increasing self-awareness. Indeed, one client wrote the following: "I tried once and found this not to be a good exercise for me. It made me too self-conscious." The reaction provided a point of discussion with the client. The client was avoiding the exercise—thinking it was not for her—because it was unsettling. But that is one of the values of the exercise. It is unsettling. It does raise the anxiety level. But these are therapeutic experiences if they are not carried to excess. I return to the poem by Burns quoted in the preface:

> Oh, would some giftie gie us
> The power to see ourselves as others see us.

It seems to me that the mirror helps you to do this to a certain extent. Try the exercise of eating in front of a mirror, and see yourself eat as others see you. It will perhaps make you self-conscious. But that is what you need to change your behavior: greater consciousness of yourself.

EAT SOMETHING WITH YOUR EYES CLOSED

The exercise called "eat something with your eyes closed" is designed to accomplish two purposes: (1) to make you more aware of the actual feeling and taste of food in your mouth, and (2) to help you realize that most of food's appeal is *visual*—not in its taste.

I thought of this exercise when I read a research report that described overweight people as *field-dependent*. That is to say that their behavior is very much controlled by external cues—the world or field about them. Internal cues—their own thoughts and ideas—tend to be subordinate to the messages coming in from the outside. (This would suggest that overweight people are more or less conforming and well-socialized in their behavior. And this appears to be true. Fat people tend not to act out their aggressions. They don't hurt others nearly as much as they hurt themselves.) This field-dependence characteristic makes it extremely difficult for overweight people to resist food at buffets, parties, etc. Seeing large amounts of food spread out on the table in a social situation creates a powerful force-field. Just as an iron filing is drawn to a magnetic field, so the overweight person is drawn to the large spread of food.

It occurred to me after reflecting on these considerations that one seldom if ever sees an overweight blind person. The blind are simply not attracted to food in the same way that people with normal vision are. Thus I reasoned that eating with the eyes closed or with a blindfold would be one way of breaking down the powerful visual association overweight persons have with food.

These are the instructions for the exercise called "eat something with your eyes closed":

Pick a time for this exercise when you are alone at home and will not be rushed. Sit down to a snack or a meal, close your eyes before eating, and eat all of the food with your eyes closed. As you eat, try to be aware of everything you experience during the eating process. After you are done eating, open your eyes and make an immediate record of your thoughts and feelings during the experiment.

Here are the reactions of a number of persons to the exercise:

"Ate cold baked beans with my eyes closed. Here are my reactions: (a) very cool refreshing feeling, (b) texture slightly rough. I like rolling them around with my tongue, (c) I can hear and feel my throat and facial muscles moving and I don't enjoy that. Normally I am not aware of the mechanics of eating, (d) I probably wouldn't enjoy foods so much if I were blind."

"I chose a chocolate pudding pie. Since I couldn't see the color, I didn't know it was dark brown, but it felt smooth and sticky, it tasted bitter, but had slight sweetness from the marshmallows and crackers. The crackers stuck to my teeth in front and sides and the marshmallow squished and felt soft. It left a bitter aftertaste, and I don't know if I would like one or not if I hadn't seen it. I think that a blind person may not like chocolate at all."

"This experience was, for me, the most interesting exercise we have done. It taught me a great many things about what kinds of 'cues' I rely upon in my eating habits. Eating with your eyes closed necessitates slowing down the entire eating process because of the difficulty of finding the food without seeing it, and finding my mouth! I suggest anyone trying this exercise use a SPOON—it is much less painful when *jammed* into your lip. Since it takes so long to eat it becomes tiresome, tedious, and rather boring. This has the effect of taking the 'fun' out of eating with me. I was forced to rely on my body cues for information, rather than external cues. When I became the slightest bit full I was more than glad to quit eating. Since I couldn't see if my plate was empty, or if the serving bowl's contents were available, I just didn't consider them in my decision to eat or to stop eating. This experiment really gave me a lot to think about in regard to the amount of attention I pay to learned cues having to do with my eating habits. I think if I listen more to *my body* I will have more success."

I think you can see from the reactions to the exercise that it can be a powerful first step in breaking down the overweight person's attraction to food on the basis of its visual appeal. The idea of the exercise is to help the overeater become more aware of his field-dependence. This awareness in turn will interfere with the smooth operation of the "see food—eat food" response pattern. However, it must be stressed that none of these exercises are effective if executed but once. A habit-breaking strategy is effective only if it is repeated many times.

DOUBLE YOUR CONSUMPTION TIME

Overeaters tend to also be fast eaters. They may think they like food, but the fact is that they almost don't taste it! It passes from their fork to the mouth to the stomach at such a rapid rate that the taste buds don't have a chance. The idea of this exercise is to encourage the overweight person to slow down and become more aware of the taste of food.

These are the instructions for the exercise:

Time yourself on how long it takes you to eat a particular item of food. Also time yourself on how long it normally takes you to eat breakfast, lunch, and dinner. Then deliberately and consciously double the amount of time you take to eat a particular food item or a particular meal. Be sure you do this *by the clock.* It is easy to kid yourself into thinking you are doubling your consumption time when in fact you may increase it by only a few minutes.

The following reactions illustrate the thoughts and feelings of persons who tried the exercise:

"During the past few weeks I've practiced the exercise. It wasn't until the beginning of the second week that I was able to comply almost 100 per cent. There were times I would become so interested in a discussion during mealtime that I'd begin to eat faster, and consequently, consumed more food. As a child I ate with forty other children in a very large dining room, and we were not permitted to utter a sound except to ask for second helpings. On one occasion the girl sitting next to me was whispering and at the same time I happened to ask for a second helping. The supervisor at the head table looked up and saw my lips moving. I was told not to talk at the table, and I replied, 'I wasn't doing the talking, I was asking for another helping.' I was told to stop sassing, and I replied that I was only sticking up for my own rights. The result was that I was placed at a table by myself in the middle of the dining room and had for my three meals for a week a bowl of bread, milk, and sugar. Don't gasp, it wasn't nearly as bad as it sounds. (The cook kept me well supplied on the side.) I only use this as an example to stress the point of why conversation today is so important to me at mealtime. I really unwind and the family opens up together. However, I can see now that the more I talk or get involved with what others are saying, I tend to consume more food than what I really need or want. Trying to double the consumption time has created a conflict because of the example stated above. But I have concentrated on it more and now find that the doubling of this consumption time is becoming less of an effort. But I can truthfully say that until this exercise was suggested I had not given previous thought to this problem."

"I found that doubling the time it normally takes me to eat something was the most helpful of the exercises—also the most difficult. At first I found myself saying, 'I just can't enjoy food when I eat so slow.' But if you really discipline yourself I can see how someone would enjoy food much more by eating slowly and making themselves more *aware* of what they're eating. Eating slowly is a habit difficult to acquire particularly if you're a nervous eater like I am—you just have to *concentrate* on slowing down—relax and try to really *taste* food for a change. It is much easier to talk about than do, though."

"I am eating a hamburger. It's really yummy. But it is kind of a funny feeling to deliberately wait between each bite. The fun of 'gorging one down' is gone. I am deeply aware of the difference."

"I ate a favorite kind of cookie while watching television and doing some studying for a midterm. Perhaps I picked a poor food for this exercise because I took one bite and put the cookie down. Waited 60 seconds (on the clock), took the second bite, repeated the process to complete the cookie. If I had chosen a larger food (cake, pie, etc.) it might have taken longer and been more effective. My attention was on the cookie all of the one and a half minutes. I felt deprived and rather ridiculous in this effort."

"Doubling the consumption time is having a positive effect on me I'm happy to say. I have to still remind myself to slow down, but miracle of miracles, it seems to be a new habit or getting there anyway. I'd rather be a 'dawdler' any day and become disinterested in food than be a gulper and never know what I'm eating. I actually find that food isn't that important *and I can slow down,* which I find gives me a sense of self-confidence. And self-confidence is rather a new phrase in my mind concerning me. I still work at this, but feel happy about the little here and there I accomplish!"

One of the reasons the overweight person eats rapidly is because he is guilty about eating. Not really tasting his food, he must go back for seconds and thirds in order to try to obtain the satisfaction from his food that he keeps missing. By slowing down and doubling the consumption time, an important step is taken in breaking down the vicious circle of eating fast, being dissatisfied, and going back for seconds and thirds.

SET A TIMER

It is fairly obvious that one of the major problems of the overeater is snacking between meals. The purpose of the exercise which follows is to provide a tool for dealing with this problem. These are the instructions:

The next time you want a snack between meals, set a timer to go off in five minutes. Do not try to use your "willpower" and say you will not snack. Just set the timer. If, when it goes off, you still want your snack, go ahead and have it. The idea of this exercise is to build up your tolerance to frustration. After you can wait five minutes, then start setting the timer for ten minutes, and so forth. You will find that you can go for longer and longer periods without snacking between meals. In time this procedure will help you completely eliminate many, if not all, between-meal snacks.

The following comments illustrate typical reactions to the "set a timer" exercise:

"After setting the timer for five minutes I decided to busy myself with housework in order to keep my mind off the food. I got so busy with my tasks that when the timer went off I kept on with what I was doing and decided not to eat at all! Bonanza, success, hooray!!! I didn't eat a thing until dinner time. I am so proud of this little success that I am eager to try it again."

"I haven't set the timer enough this past week and I have nibbled and picked. This is really a bad habit, and it is going to take a lot of self-discipline. I find I'm nibbling (a piece of pie is nibbling??!) without thinking of the timer, but because I neglected this and see its *real* importance, this exercise will be foremost in my mind. I get angry when I think about it—if I wasn't such a weakling I wouldn't need this 'gimmick.' Damn, this makes me *mad!*"

"Tried this exercise and found this to be the best exercise for me. When I would put a five-minute time on something I wanted to eat I would forget about the food in that time and be doing something else—maybe an hour or two hours later remember that I had wanted to nibble."

"The timer worked! I only nibbled once during the week and this was because someone bought me some popcorn (and I don't like popcorn that well)."

"Setting the timer gave me a chance to think and reflect about my behavior. During the time delay I would think, 'Do I really want this snack? Do I really want to stay fat?' I would become very conscious of my behavior, and would often find the desire to snack gone when the timer went off. I followed instructions and had a snack if the desire was still there. But this happened less than half of the time. I'm working on extending the delay to fifteen minutes now. When I'm not at home I use my watch as a timer—but find this doesn't work as well as when I can actually 'set' something."

As you can see from these quotations, reactions to the "set a timer" exercise are fairly consistent. Some people find it very difficult to do the exercise—they resist it. But if the timer is actually set and a decision is made to make the five-minute wait, then the majority of persons report beneficial results from the exercise. These persons say that the desire for a snack is gone when the timer goes off—or they forget all about wanting to snack when they busy themselves with something else during the delay period.

Although the exercise may sound both simple and superficial, there are deeper implications. Assuming that much of an overeater's behavior consists of well-established bad habits, we are forced to also assume that the overeater is not thinking when he nibbles or takes a snack. He does it in a half-conscious fashion. Certainly he is not reflecting on his behavior. Once again we have a case of conditioning, a "stimulus-response" connection as psychologists put it. The sequence is: see food—eat food. Thought and reflection have dropped out of the picture. But thought and reflection are the basic elements in human freedom. Thought and reflection permit us to change bad habits. Thus, setting the timer for even five minutes sets up the following sequence: see food . . . thought and reflection . . . behavior alternatives other than eating. The smooth execution of the habit is destroyed by the opportunity to think which takes place during the delay period. In terms of neurophysiology we would say that setting the timer gives a chance for your neocortex to get into the picture. The neocortex is the "new brain"—the part of your brain that makes you a human being—an aware organism. So give your "new brain" a chance. Set the timer and let the time delay interfere with the semiautomatic habit of snacking between meals.

LIST ALL OF THE THINGS YOU CAN DO WITH A COOKIE

The general principle behind all of these habit-breaking exercises is the idea of increasing the general consciousness of your own behavior and your relationship to food. In line with this principle we might say that the overweight person has one simple relationship with food—he eats it. The purpose of the following exercise is to attempt to look at food differently—to develop a perspective and a flexibility toward food not possessed by the average overeater. It can be a valuable exercise to deliberately try to perceive food as something other than an object of consumption.

Think of this as an exercise in creativity. Place a cookie (or other desirable food) before you. Now look at it, think about it, but don't eat it. Try to think of all the things you can do with a cookie other than the rather obvious act of eating it. Be as flexible and imaginative in your thinking as possible. Close your eyes and let images come to mind. Make a list of all of the things that occur to you. Should you eat the cookie at the end of the exercise? That's up to you. Don't try to use your "willpower" to resist it—but observe if your desire for the cookie has changed in some subtle way.

Here are some reactions to the exercise:

"Uses for a cookie: (1) decorate and use as a Christmas tree ornament, (2) shape into figure and arrange a table centerpiece around it, (3) use one for a medallion around your neck, (4) write your name on it in frosting and use it as a place mark, (5) make a heart-shaped one for a valentine. At the end of a meal I took one bite of a cookie and gave it away—surprised, I realized I wasn't really hungry."

"What to do with your spare uneaten cookies: (1) use four of them for hub caps on your mini car, (2) use them for buttons on a dress, (3) use them for earrings, (4) make an abacus with cookies to replace the beads, (5) use them for money instead of coins in a telephone booth, (6) make yourself a cookie bookmark, (7) put one over your left eye and run for prime minister of Israel, (8) put them on the record player and hear the latest hits, (9) patch a hole in your shoe with cookies, (10) paint a peace symbol on it and hang it around your neck, (11) use them for handles on cabinets, (12) use them for checkers in your next game, (13) paint numbers on one and use it for a watch, (14) build a doll house made of cookies, (15) build a wall with Fig Newtons to go around your doll house made of cookies, (16) create a piece of artwork and frame it, (17) mark all your favorite cities on the map with cookies, (18) use them for tokens on the Staten Island ferry. I have invested so much of my libido into this list that I have lost all desire for a cookie. Who wants to eat a cookie when there are so many creative things to do in this world? Only unimaginative boors eat cookies!!!"

"What to do with a cookie besides eating it: (1) crumble it for the birds, (2) decorate and hang on Xmas tree, (3) decorate and use it for a place marker at a dinner, (4) soak in milk and feed it to a baby, (5) sell it as Campfire Girls do, (6) use it for a paperweight, (7) use it for bait to catch a mouse, (8) give it to children on Halloween, (9) leave it in the cupboard for the ants, (10) hang it on a string to form a mobile, (11) use it for a collage. After writing out these exercises I took the cookie off the plate (I had placed it on a plate on the table before me while thinking up things to do) and I put it back in the cookie jar. I haven't had a desire to eat a cookie for two weeks."

The following reaction was given by one client to a different food, ice cream: "What can I do with ice cream? Let it melt and get warm, then try to eat it—ugh—can't do it! Can't eat that warm mess! Imagine finger painting with it—just sloshing it all over paper, table and everywhere—yuk! I wouldn't eat finger paint. Smear it all over my face. I hate this. Let it dry on my hands—no! I shudder at all these things. (Sticky mess!) I fantasize myself eating ice cream *all* day long, nothing else and I almost become physically ill. It is a hot day, I am bushed. But instead of going swimming in the pool, I will dive into a great vat of all my (formerly) favorite flavors of ICE CREAM! It is a nightmare. I am not soothed with the coolness. I am smothered by the sweet, gooey mess. I get half-ill at the sight or thought of ice cream."

You may be dubious that the exercise of writing out all of the things you can do with a particular food item can have the effects reported. I suggest you give it a try and find out for yourself. Don't refer to the lists given in this book, of course. It would probably be better to try the exercise with foods other than a cookie or ice cream. You obviously will get the greatest benefit if the ideas and images that come to mind are your own. Try the exercise with those favorite foods that give you a problem: pie, cake, bread, potato chips, french fries, nuts, etc.

BAKE SOMETHING AND GIVE IT AWAY

The behavioristic psychologist Edwin Guthrie used to say that if you want to break a habit, "Practice a different response to the stimulus." In this case the stimulus is food. The purpose of the exercise described below is the same as the previous exercises: to make you more aware of your eating habits, to make your behavior more flexible. By deliberately and consciously practicing a different response to food than the familiar one (eating it), you begin to break up your stereotyped habit patterns.

The instructions for the exercise called "bake something and give it away" follow:

Bake one of your favorite high-carbohydrate desserts (e.g., a cake, a pie, cookies, etc.). Then make a gift of the dessert to a friend, relative, or neighbor. It is very important that you look at, smell, and experience the food item in every way *except eating it*. When you give the food item away, do not then figure it is all right to have a piece. The idea is to give it *all* away. You are not to eat any of it.

Here are some reactions to the exercise:

"I baked brownies this week and gave them to my grandparents. I felt very good about this. Plus by baking something chocolate it made me want it more. But I just said to myself, 'I hate chocolate,' and then I didn't want the item. I don't need chocolate for my complexion."

"I baked a chocolate cake and gave it to my next-door neighbor. This made me really proud of myself; I felt so good. I forgot it as soon as it was gone."

"I have had no opportunity to bake something this past week. My husband has been gone, working from 4 P.M. to 12 A.M., and I have been at my exam studies. This won't be too difficult for me, though. I can do this and by giving the item away I get the reward of the pleasure received from those to whom I give it." (Author's note: Client's comment may indicate both resistance toward the exercise and rationalization about not doing it. Nevertheless, the comment is still of value to a therapist. If the client is resisting and rationalizing, these are things that need to be worked through. The therapist can test the level of her resistance by asking her to do the assignment the following week, again requesting a written reaction describing thoughts and feelings.)

"This week I made a gorgeous, fattening batch of German chocolate brownies with gooey frosting. What a sense of power!! No bowl licking or finger dipping either! I cut the whole batch into squares and put them on a plate. (They were *so* moist—funny, they never turn out as good when I make them for my own feasting!) I took them over to this fellow I've been dating and he sat and ate three of them *right in front of me!* But seriously, when I started fixing them I was very aware of the fact that 'these are not for me' and this made the whole deal much easier."

Here is a reaction from a male client:

"I like to putter around in the kitchen, and I figured I'd make an instant cake. I cooked it one evening after work and I took it to the office the next day for coffee break. It all went. I didn't have a bite and some of the girls in the office got a big kick out of it when I explained why I had done it. However, I doubt that this could serve as a regular habit-breaking device for a man. You get kidded too much. But the exercise was valuable to me. I did learn something from it. I learned that your 'mental set' or initial attitude toward food has a lot to do with whether or not you're going to eat it. My intention was not to eat the cake, and I didn't! A good feeling!"

Here are two reactions from a patient named Mary K:

(First reaction): "I baked a birthday cake for Doris. But even after making what I considered to be a firm decision not to eat any, I broke down and ate one-half piece. Damn! No self-control! (Sure tasted good though.)"

(Second reaction): "I baked banana nut bread—drool, drool, drool and gave it to my next-door neighbor. My self-control was high at this time so I didn't feel too bad. My worst moments were while the bread was baking. The anticipation of the taste, the odor wafting through the kitchen, and the sight of it nearly got me!"

As you can see from the above reactions, baking something and giving it away is a fairly difficult exercise. But, of course, its value resides in this very fact. Recall what was said about classical conditioning in Chapter 4. In order for extinction to occur one must remain in the presence of the conditioned stimuli without reinforcement. Mary's second reaction in which she says "the anticipation of the taste, the odor wafting through the kitchen, and the sight of it nearly got me!" is a good example of a deconditioning experience. By exposing herself to the conditioned stimuli (the odor of the bread, the sight of the bread) *without eating it* she took a large step toward breaking her dependence upon food.

ANALYZE YOUR TASTE SENSATIONS

I have said before that the most overweight people don't really taste their food. They gobble. The food is usually half-chewed. They are thinking of the second helping while eating the first helping. They think they like food—many fat people think of themselves as food gourmets. But a real gourmet *tastes* his food—he really experiences it fully. As a habit-breaking technique to counteract this tendency it can be very helpful to make a food graph of some favorite foods. The idea of the food graph is derived from the work of the father of experimental psychology, Wilhelm Wundt. Wundt is the one who proposed, on the basis of his experiments, that all food tastes could be broken down into four basic sensations: sweet, sour, bitter, and salty. The idea of the exercise which follows is to make a conscious effort to analyze your taste experience of a particular food into its sensory elements. The exercise will help you become a gourmet instead of a glutton. Here are the basic instructions:

Select a favorite food. Do this exercise when you are alone and have plenty of time. You are going to pretend that you are a taster for a big food company. It is your job to analyze the food item into its basic elements. This is to be a quantitative analysis—we need to know the magnitude of each taste sensation. In order to help you make the analysis, use the following graph:

Sweet	0	1	2	3	4	5	6	7	8	9	10
Sour	0	1	2	3	4	5	6	7	8	9	10
Bitter	0	1	2	3	4	5	6	7	8	9	10
Salty	0	1	2	3	4	5	6	7	8	9	10

Circle the number that most closely represents the magnitude of the particular sensation. For example, if the food item has no sweetness at all, circle the zero. If it has just a grace of sweetness, circle the 1, and so forth. After you have decided how sweet the food item is, then make a decision about the sour, bitter, and salty sensations. Connect the circles with straight lines, and you now have a graphic portrayal of your taste analysis of a particular food. Do this with a number of foods, and also record your reactions to the exercise.

Here are some reactions to the experiment:

"The food I decided to analyze was beer. I'm not sure that beer is a 'food'—but I know it's fattening and has food value. So I decided to analyze it.

BEER ANALYSIS

Sweet	⓪	1	2	3	4	5	6	7	8	9	10
Sour	⓪	1	2	3	4	5	6	7	8	9	10
Bitter	0	1	2	③	4	5	6	7	8	9	10
Salty	0	1	②	3	4	5	6	7	8	9	10

Do you know what you're going to do? You're going to take all the fun of drinking beer away—but I guess that's the idea isn't it? No, I don't mean that. My reaction to the experiment is mixed—it was hard to do. I keep looking at the graph and thinking, 'But there must be more to the taste of beer than that.' The graph looks so thin—all I'm getting out of beer is just a little bitterness and saltiness."

"I'm a meat and potatoes man, and my favorite meal out is a broiled steak and a baked potato loaded with sour cream. I decided to analyze the taste of a steak.

STEAK ANALYSIS

	0	1	2	3	4	5	6	7	8	9	10
Sweet	0	1	(2)	3	4	5	6	7	8	9	10
Sour	(0)	1	2	3	4	5	6	7	8	9	10
Bitter	(0)	1	2	3	4	5	6	7	8	9	10
Salty	0	1	2	3	(4)	5	6	7	8	9	10

After looking at the graph and thinking about the experience of analyzing the taste, I'm beginning to realize that I don't eat for taste at all. There's just not that much taste there when you sit down to analyze it. The experience of analyzing the taste of steak has really helped me to slow down. I'm eating food and *trying* to taste it—maybe for the first time. And it's hard to do. It's a real effort to actually *taste* food."

"I've always been crazy about burritos. I know they're fattening. So I decided to analyze the taste of a burrito.

BURRITO ANALYSIS

	0	1	2	3	4	5	6	7	8	9	10
Sweet	(0)	1	2	3	4	5	6	7	8	9	10
Sour	0	(1)	2	3	4	5	6	7	8	9	10
Bitter	(0)	1	2	3	4	5	6	7	8	9	10
Salty	0	(1)	2	3	4	5	6	7	8	9	10

This is incredible! Is that all the taste I can get out of a burrito? I can certainly see how this exercise ties in with the exercise of eating with your eyes closed. I'm beginning to realize that the fat person is much more hooked on *how food looks* than how it tastes. But when you realize that you can *look* at food all you want without gaining an ounce, you begin to wonder why you have to eat it. Overeating is ridiculous. Why not just look at food, enjoy its appearance, and eat some of it slowly. When you've had enough, just stop! You don't have to lick the platter clean every time like I've been doing."

I could present a number of other reactions. But the general response to this exercise is fairly uniform. The overweight person recognizes with a mild shock that he hasn't really been tasting his food. And he also recognizes that taste sensations are not intense sensations. Our experience of a food is really a total experience involving not only taste sensations. All of our senses are involved when we eat. We see the food—its appearance is of great importance. We smell the food; the smell of food is as important as its taste. You have probably heard that when a person is blindfolded and holds his nose it is hard to tell an onion from a potato. (Try it if you don't believe it.) Touch is important in a food experience. Certainly the difference in texture between french fries and mashed potatoes is an important part of the difference we experience between them. And our ability to discriminate textures is because of the sense of touch. The sense of touch exists in your mouth as much as it does in your finger. And even hearing can't be left out. When we crunch down on a potato chip we hear it snap. We hear the sizzle of a steak. The important point is that all of these experiences are *nonfattening*. If you slow down, you can have them all—like a gourmet— without eating a great amount. The amount of food you eat doesn't increase the intensity of these experiences. Quite the contrary—it decreases them. By eating fast you *miss* the total experience—you don't give yourself a chance to attend to and notice the many sensations it is possible to experience when you eat.

But don't just resolve to slow down. Actually do the food analysis exercise. Analyze a number of your favorite fattening foods. You will find yourself slowing down with very little difficulty as you make the analysis. Your effort to taste the food—really taste it—will inhibit your tendency to eat rapidly. It will be an interesting experience. If you do the exercise a number of times over a period of several weeks, you will find the tendency to slow down and taste your food generalizes to other eating situations. By doing the taste analysis experiment you will become aware of how important all of your senses are in the experience of eating.

THE EYEBALLING SATIATION TECHNIQUE

I hope we agree by now that the overweight person is very much controlled by food as a visual stimulus. He sees food and this makes him hungry. When he looks through a magazine with photographs of well-prepared foods, he can become excited and feel food-deprived. How can you decondition yourself to food as a visual stimulus? I think that many overweight people make a serious mistake. They try to hide food from themselves. All the cookies, nuts, ice cream, etc., are hidden away in cupboards and the refrigerator. Housewives who have to stay alone in the house for hours with young children often have a problem with between-meal snacking. A common "gimmick" that is used is to stick a sign on the refrigerator door that says, "Don't pick!" or "Don't be a pig!" I think it would be a far better idea to stick a picture of some delicious food on the door of the refrigerator. Look at the picture to your heart's content. You will find that soon the picture will become meaningless—it will lose its attraction and its ability to excite you. Do this with a number of photographs. You will find yourself less and less aroused by the sheer sight of food.

In line with this general concept I formulated the following exercise called "the eyeballing satiation technique."

As usual, pick a time when you are alone for this exercise. Take a favorite item of food (e.g., a piece of candy). Place it on a plate. Now sit down and *by the clock* stare at it for five minutes. Whether or not you eat it at the end of the five minutes is irrelevant to the exercise. Don't try to use "will-power." The idea is to see how you feel about the food after staring at it for five minutes. Record your thoughts and feelings.

Here are some reactions to the exercise:

"I stared at a piece of candy for five minutes. At first it looked delicious, and I thought I would only be able to look at it for about a half of a minute—and then I figured I would have to eat it. But after about a minute something peculiar seemed to happen to my perception. The candy seemed to *shrink*. That's right! It looked smaller on the plate somehow. I can't explain it. But I got so fascinated by this 'illusion' that I continued to stare at the candy to see what would happen next. Suddenly it seemed to expand back to its normal size. I don't mean that I was having a hallucination or anything. I didn't think the candy was actually shrinking or expanding. It was strictly a perceptual thing. But it was fascinating. It must have something to do with staring in the same direction and fixating on the same object. Anyway, after a few minutes the candy seemed to lose some of its attractiveness as food. At the end of the five minutes I replaced it in the candy box with no problem. I didn't really want to eat it."

"I tried this exercise with a hamburger and french fries. There's a coffee shop on my way home, and almost every day

I stop in and order a hamburger plate with french fries. You have to understand that this is 'sneak eating.' Right after I leave the coffee shop I drive home, and no more than an hour later my wife is serving dinner. I tried the eyeballing satiation technique with the hamburger plate the last time I stopped in. I ordered the plate, and when it came I determined to myself that I was just going to sit there and look at it for five solid minutes before I ate it. I don't know what I expected. I certainly didn't expect my desire for the food to go away. But the most peculiar thing happened. As I looked at the food I began thinking, 'Why am I doing this? Why do I want this stuff? Do I really want to keep looking like a hog all my life?' I began rethinking some of the reasons I overeat and what food means to me. By the end of the five minutes the food looked like THE ENEMY. I had no desire to eat it at all. It was just a cold hamburger and greasy fries that would make me fatter and more uncomfortable. I got up, paid my check at the cashier, and left without a word of explanation. The food remained on the table. And I haven't been back to that coffee shop all week. And the funny part of it is I don't want to stop there or anywhere else for a hamburger or french fries."

"I tried the exercise with ice cream. I guess this was kind of unfair because I knew that by the end of five minutes the melted ice cream might not appeal to me. But I tried it anyway. Actually, the ice cream was still pretty hard at the end of five minutes. And I still wanted it. So I ate it. But even then the exercise somehow did something to my desire for ice cream. I wouldn't want any now. For some reason it's not appealing."

"Candy is my downfall. The kind you get from the candy machine at work. I got out a candy bar and took it with me on my coffee break. I usually gobble it up with a couple of cups of coffee. This time I unwrapped it and placed it on the table during the break. I didn't explain to the other girls what I was doing or why. I just let the candy stay there on the wrapper as I sipped my coffee. I was very very aware of it. But the other girls didn't even seem to notice what I was doing. Funny, something that's a big thing to you is nothing to someone else. Anyway, at the end of five minutes the candy had just lost its appeal. I didn't know what to do with it. I knew I wasn't going to eat it. I casually offered it to one of the other girls, saying that I just didn't want it. She took it with good cheer—not even puzzled by my buying it and not eating it. She's thin, I might note. I watched what she did with the candy. She ate half of it, and when our break was over she threw about half of the candy bar into the trash. I would have never done that with something someone else gave me. But I'm just beginning to realize that thin people don't value food the way I do. To them it's just something else. They can take it or leave it. This is so obvious that it's riciculous to even write it down. And yet it seems to be dawning on me for the first time. Anyway, the exercise was a good one and I think it helped me. I'll try it again with pecan pie next."

"It took me three weeks to try this exercise. I know, I know—resistance! All the more reason I should do the exer ise—right? So I finally got up the gumption to do it with a piece of leftover birthday cake. In our house I'm the one who usually polishes off all the leftovers. My family doesn't like leftovers, and I think they're yummy. In this case it was my son's birthday cake. The time of the 'great experiment' was 10:00 A.M. I fixed myself a cup of coffee, cut a slice of cake, and sat down all by myself at the kitchen table. My mind was filled with rationalizations, 'I need the energy. After all, I'm going to vacuum today.' But I was determined to stare at the cake for five minutes before I ate it. So I stared at it. I really looked at it. I studied the frosting, and suddenly I thought, 'That's sugar and shortening. That's all it is.' Suddenly it wasn't 'frosting' anymore. It was sugar and shortening. Then I looked at the cake itself. It was crumbly and moist. But I began thinking, 'What is it? Just sugar, shortening, and flour. Carbohydrates, pure carbohydrates.' The thing seemed to deteriorate before my eyes from an appealing cake to just a bunch of sugar and lard in that short span of time. I didn't know what to do with the cake. I wanted to throw it away down the garbage disposal. But that seemed wrong. So I put it back into the cake dish. No one in the household ate it. So in a few days it was stale, and it ended up in the trash anyway. I felt guilty throwing the food into the trash knowing how overpopulated the world is and how many people don't have enough to eat. But this has made me all the more determined not to be a glutton and overeat. I'm certainly not helping the starving people of the world by overeating. Eating that cake wouldn't have helped them one bit. It should certainly be possible for us to *not* overeat and *not* waste food."

The reactions to the eyeballing satiation technique indicate that something happens to food's appeal if you study it carefully for a time before you eat it. You satiate on its appearance. It loses its capacity to excite you. You may not get this effect the first time you try the exercise. But ry it more than once. If you end up eating the food item, it indicates that you need quite a bit of deconditioning experience to break the hold that food has over you.

The most common objection voiced about the habit-breaking exercises discussed in this chapter is, "But isn't overeating a problem with unconscious emotional roots? Aren't these habit-breaking exercises a superficial approach?"

From what I have said in previous chapters, I think you

can see that I agree with the premise that the overweight person has to learn to deal effectively with his unconscious motives and his ego defense mechanisms. However, that does not mean that the problem of chronic overeating is entirely emotional and ego defensive. Even if the underlying personality structure of the overweight person is altered in a positive direction, he is left with the residual effects of poor eating habits. For example, let us say that you normally write with your right hand. Assume that your right hand is badly injured in an accident, and it is essential that you learn how to write with your left hand. Pick up a pen or pencil and write your name with your left hand. See how difficult it is. You can barely do it. Even if you no longer had the use of your right hand, the first time you used your left hand for writing, you would experience this difficulty. The only way you could learn to use your left hand effectively would be by a great deal of practice. You would consciously and deliberately have to overcome old habit tendencies in order to get the new habit established. Would this difficulty be the result of unconscious motives and ego defense mechanisms? Would this difficulty be "resistance to therapy?" I doubt it. Obviously, you have to go through a period of clumsiness whenever you learn something new or change a well-established habit pattern. In the same manner, an overweight person has to overcome years of responding to food in a stereotyped manner. The purpose of the exercises presented in this chapter is to give you a way of putting some "static" between the stimulus of food and your habitual responses to it.

Look at it this way: we all experience frustration, anxiety, and depression. Many overweight persons may experience no more frustration, anxiety, and depression than the "normal" person. But the normal person has devised a number of flexible strategies for dealing with his emotional conflicts.

One person may be an amateur writer and displace hostility by writing murder mysteries. Another person may have a punching bag in the garage and get rid of anger by hitting the bag around. Still another person may paint pictures of monsters as a harmless way of expressing the "monsters" on the inside (i.e., "hang-ups," conflicts, etc.). These are all healthy outlets and tend to drain off the power of negative emotions. But the chronic overeater has fallen into the doldrums. Negative emotions produce a yearning for food, and a raid on the refrigerator is called for.

Although it is essential to understand one's emotional life, it is also essential to develop flexible strategies for dealing with negative emotions when they occur. And it is also essential to break up the stereotyped pattern of overeating as the favorite way of dealing with negative emotions. Practice the exercises outlined in this chapter, and start to break up your undesirable eating habits.

Chapter 6
Creative Weight Control

What is creativity? The essence of creativity is *novelty*. A creative solution to an old problem implies a novel and previously unexamined approach to the problem. For example, when Albert Einstein put his mind to dealing with certain problems arising in physics due to apparent contradictions, he "solved" the problem by deciding that time can slow down in certain situations and space can warp in other situations. This was certainly a novel solution to the problems of physics. The great Sir Isaac Newton had stated that space had absolute extensity and time flowed at a constant rate throughout the universe. It was a breakthrough in thinking to reject these "obvious" truths.

Many of us like to think of ourselves as creative. But how many of us have attempted to solve our weight problems by novel, and nonobvious strategies? I think that too often when the overweight person tries to lose weight he *does not* diet creatively. He goes on a diet with an attitude of martyrdom. His attitude is one of self-sacrifice and self-pity. The whole attitude is one of "When can I get off of the diet?" Instead of approaching the weight loss program with a spirit of creativity and adventure, an opportunity for new experience, most individuals are cast immediately into the psychological doldrums by the very thought of dieting.

Remember once again that losing weight is in fact a process that—if it is to be successful—involves *relearning.* Psychologists have discovered a great deal about human learning. There are certain basic principles that should not be ignored. Most of these are well established, and they are well accepted by the psychological community. However, most psychology textbooks obviously do not make a systematic attempt to apply these principles to the problem of the overweight person. In this chapter, we attempt to do this. The creative dieting suggestions that follow are based on these sound psychological principles. I will in each case attempt to identify the principle involved. I think of these suggestions as *creative dieting* because so often they involve strategies that have not occurred to most overweight people.

KEEP A DIET DIARY

One of the most valuable suggestions I have made for some overweight people is to *keep a diet diary.* The principle involved here is the one of *making yourself more conscious of your behavior.* This is much like Knight Dunlap's principle of negative practice cited in Chapter 5.

I am including portions from one client's diary in order to illustrate what a diary is like. The writer is a twenty-eight-year-old homemaker. Her husband is struggling to establish himself as a life insurance salesman. She spends many days and evenings without adult companionship caring for an infant and a toddler. She is a well-educated, licensed teacher, but she has not worked in her profession for five years:

MONDAY

This is the first entry in my diet diary. Dr. Bruno says this will make me more conscious of exactly what is going on in my struggle to lose weight. I weighed myself this morning, and I weighed 188 pounds. I want to weigh 125. I'm so angry at myself for overeating Saturday night at the wedding and overeating Sunday at the family get-together.

For lunch I had two wieners and sauerkraut. No breakfast this morning because I felt stuffed from yesterday. My desire to lose weight is very strong today. Very strong. And yet I've found that you can gain weight even when your desire to lose it is very strong. It's the presence of food—seeing the damn food right out there in front of you that does it.

Right now I'm having a glass of skim milk. I think I'll make that my afternoon snack from now on. Milk is great for your nerves. Going to try and cut out the coffee. Not so much coffee from now on. I know that coffee triggers the desire to eat. I used to drink coffee to have something oral to do while not eating. But now I wonder.

TUESDAY

You have to think—*really think*—about your overeating. Why you do it, when you do it, how you do it. I can see that writing this out is a way of taking thought chains and carrying them through to conclusions. It is *not* a matter of thinking before you write—you have to think *as* you write. If we want to learn a poem it is better to recite it aloud. If we want to learn to drive a car, it is better to drive a car than to just sit and think about driving a car. And if we want to think things through we need to think aloud, so to speak. This is what bull sessions are—group therapy, etc. And this self-analysis is another way of accomplishing the same thing. Also, it moves the problem to the *center* of my consciousness.

WEDNESDAY

I'm not going to weigh myself every day. Too much. I'm going to weigh once a week. I'm becoming a slave to the scale.

I'm thinking that people think negatively about dieting. They figure, "Oh, what's the use? Even if I get it off I'll never keep it off." That's what they think way down deep. Okay—get that thought right out here on paper into the center of your conscious mind. Here is a counter thought: You won't necessarily gain back the weight you lose. I think I can do it. I know I can do it.

THURSDAY

Well, my motivational level remains high. Although I see I have a tendency to put this off. However, this is the first chance I've really had today to get to it (2:00 P.M.). For breakfast I had an egg and toast. For lunch I had salad with vinegar and oil, baked fish—did not eat tartar sauce—just squeezed lemon juice on it. I had plain steamed cauliflower. Tonight I intend to have a steak, salad, and a vegetable. For my afternoon snack I'll have a glass of skim milk. Tomorrow morning I'll have one of these: glass of skim milk, beef patty, or egg again.

FRIDAY

Yesterday afternoon I ate a piece of chicken—stripped off the skin. But I really think that was a slip because I had said that I wasn't going to have a food snack—just a glass of skim milk. I think it's really hard to suppress my oral needs. Right now they don't seem so strong. Had a light but satisfying lunch. Roast turkey without the dressing, salad with just vinegar—got some oil on it by mistake, and peas. Okay—what is my intention for this afternoon? Just a glass of skim milk—no coffee. Hey, there's a bona find insight. (Meant to say *fide*—not *find*—it is a "find" when you have an insight.) Hey, I really feel good about this!

KEEP A WEIGHT LOSS GRAPH

This creative dieting suggestion is called *keep a weight loss graph.* It is based on the principle of *feedback* or *knowledge of results.* One of the most well-established principles in human learning and human motivation is the principle of *feedback.* You need to know the results of your performance. If, for example, you were learning to type, and you could not see the results of your work, it would take you a very long time to learn to become an efficient typist. And you would lose all of your motivation. For a moment postulate the absurdity of learning to type without a typewriter ribbon and without paper in the typewriter. You couldn't tell if you were making mistakes or not. There would be no way to judge your work. It would obviously be nonsense to try to teach people to type without a ribbon or without paper. Let's take one more absurd example just to make the point. Let's say you were learning to shoot a bow and arrow. Do you think you would ever learn if you were made to practice with a blindfold? Of course not. So it's glaringly obvious that feedback or knowledge of results is essential to learning.

As you are losing weight, you are learning. You are learning to understand yourself, and you are learning new eating habits. Therefore, you should take advantage of the principle of feedback. One of the ways you can do this is by weighing yourself regularly and keeping a weight loss graph.

Along the horizontal axis of your graph, mark off a *time line*. For example: January 1, 2, 3, 4, etc. Along the vertical axis of the graph mark off pounds. At the top of the vertical axis place your present weight. For example, if your present weight is 180 pounds, write 180 pounds at the top of the graph. For each space below that put one pound less: 179, 178, 177, etc. Now you can plot your weight loss as a decreasing function of time.

One of the really interesting things you can do with a weight loss graph is to place on the graph a *trend line* which shows your predicted weight loss—what you expect to do. Be realistic about this. Let's say that you feel you can lose two pounds a week. Mark in a trend line showing a two-pound loss per week. Then you can plot the actual record of your weight loss against this predicted trend line. This will give you a vivid visual display of either your failure or success with your dieting efforts. It can be quite motivating to try to match the predicted trend line. Also, another advantage of this procedure is that if you find yourself falling sharply below your predicted trend line you can grant yourself a food indulgence from time to time without feeling guilty. After all, all you are asking of yourself is to match the trend line. On the other hand, if you find yourself staying above the trend line, this will motivate you to exercise somewhat greater efforts in controlling your intake of food.

I have found keeping the weight loss graph a very helpful strategy. It helps to give your dieting efforts a structure. Like keeping the diary it makes you more conscious of your eating patterns, and all in all it can be a device which at the same time helps both your motivation and your learning of new eating patterns. I encourage you to try it.

THE ON-OFF APPROACH

Learning proceeds best under conditions of distributed practice rather than under conditions of massed practice. When we practice something continuously we get bored, fatigued, and our attention wanders. In order to illustrate the operation of this fundamental principle, let's pretend that we're doing a human learning experiment with children. The children are being asked to learn the pathway of a complex pencil maze—one of those mazes where the child has to work his way out from the center tracing his path with a pencil. You are probably familiar with this kind of maze from children's books and comic strips.

In this experiment the children are divided into two groups. One group is called the experimental group. The other group is called the control group. The control group receives massed practice. They have ten opportunities to learn the maze, and all ten practice sessions occur one right after the other in the same afternoon. The other group, the experimental group, receives only one practice session per day. They practice once a day for ten days. The second group—the experimental group—has received *distributed practice*. But note that *both groups* have received the same total amount of practice. Which group fares better on a "final exam" that involves a measure of the number of errors a subject makes in completing the maze, and the amount of time required to escape from the maze? The answer is that the experimental group, the group that received distributed practice, does far, far better than the group that received massed practice. This shows quite clearly that the experimental group got much more out of its practice sessions because of the fact that its members were able to practice with less chance of becoming bored and fatigued.

You can take advantage of the beneficial effects of distributed practice as a form of creative dieting. For example, whoever said that when you are dieting you have to be on a diet every day? It can be very discouraging to feel that you are dieting every day. So a simple strategy that could be adopted is to diet *every other day*. For example, you might diet Monday, Wednesday, Friday, and Sunday. Then you could go off your diet on Tuesday, Thursday, and Saturday. This would give you four days on and three days off. You will find it much easier to stick to your diet on your "on" days because you can look forward to your "off" days. Remember, it is the *total amount* of calories or carbohydrates consumed that counts. The amounts you consume on individual days are of little importance. If, for example, you have determined that you can lose weight on 1200 calories a day, you could arrange your diet in such a way that on your "on" days you consume only 600 or 700 calories. These would be days of semifasting. And on your "off" days you could consume as many as 1800 calories. As a consequence of following this strategy, you would not have to eliminate entirely from your diet various kinds of treats. There are many benefits to this kind of a strategy. As an illustration, you do not feel so sorry for yourself. You have something to look forward to. It is possible to maintain your diet on your "on" days because you have the freedom of the "off" days.

Many people, when they go on a diet, feel they must always be on the diet. Consequently, if they have a cookie or a piece of cake, they feel that they have broken the diet, they have failed, and they throw all caution to the winds and go completely off the diet. I think this is an example of the kind of oversimplified black-white thinking that often gets us into trouble. We oversimplify, we expect too much of ourselves. It is almost unreasonable to expect that an individual who has a taste for sweets or rich foods will simply cut them out totally and completely from his diet once and for all until he achieves a normal weight.

You may find that the on-off every other day pattern is not the best one for you. There are all kinds of on-off patterns. One woman client recently devised the following pattern: four days on the diet and one day off the diet. Then she went back on the diet again for four days, and then off again for one day. This made her off day fall on rotating days of the week. For example, let's say that she started her diet on Monday. So she dieted Monday, Tuesday, Wednesday, and Thursday. Then she went off her diet on Friday. Then she went back on her diet Saturday, Sunday, Monday, and Tuesday. She then went off her diet again on Wednesday. And so forth. This kept changing the day of the week she could go off her diet, and created a novel pattern. One of the interesting things about this strategy as she reported it to me was that when it came for the day that she could go off her diet, she often did not in fact feel like overindulging herself. Nevertheless, the fact that she had the *freedom* to go off her diet *without guilt* was very important. She did not feel sorry for herself nor terribly deprived during her four diet days because she knew she had the "off" day to look forward to if she wanted it. This woman as of this writing lost more than twenty pounds using this four days on and one day off strategy. She weighed more than 190 pounds when she started losing weight, and this is the first substantial weight loss she has had in more than twenty years.

As I have already indicated, the on-off strategy is based on very sound and well-established principles of learning and motivation. Work out an on-off pattern that appeals to you, and give it a try. I think you'll be pleasantly surprised with the results.

SET SUBGOALS

When a goal is very far away it is sometimes hard to get excited about it. It is so far away that the attainment of it seems almost impossible. This is a psychological principle sometimes called the *goal-gradient hypothesis*. It was formulated by the behavioristic psychologist Clark L. Hull in his book *Principles of Behavior*. If you'll pardon for a moment a reference to an experiment with rats, Hull found that rats learn mazes *backwards*. They ran faster in the maze when they were near their goal—the food placed at the end of the maze by Hull or his assistants. They also eliminated errors from the goal area back to the starting box; that is to say, that when an animal began learning the maze and stopped going into blind alleys the animals stopped going into blind alleys near the goal *first*. In other words, they learned the maze backwards. This indicates that when organisms are near a goal they are both more motivated and they learn more rapidly. Of course, this experiment was done with rats. And perhaps we shouldn't be too quick to generalize to human beings. However, if the basic principles of learning are the same for all organisms—and some psychologists seem to think they are—then the experiment is applicable.

Let's simply approach it on a commonsense level. When is a student more likely to drop out of college? When he is a freshman with four years to go? Or when he is a senior with perhaps only a semester left before he attains his B.A. degree? It is perfectly obvious that an individual who has only a small amount left to go in college is both more motivated and more attentive to what he needs to learn. This is the *goal-gradient hypothesis* in action in human affairs. I don't really think we need to resort to the rat experiment to establish the validity of the goal-gradient hypothesis. It seems perfectly obvious to me that when you are near your goals you are more motivated and more likely to maintain your goal-directed behavior.

How does this apply to the individual who is trying to lose weight? Let us assume that the overweight person has a long way to go before he or she will be a normal weight. One client, Mrs. Alice Z., weighed 200 pounds. In order to be a normal weight she would have to be as little as 125 pounds. A weight loss of seventy pounds looked so formidable to her that she was completely discouraged and could not even start to diet. So we set a subgoal for her. We established a new "ideal" weight. Temporarily she was to think of 180 pounds as an ideal weight. She was not to think beyond this. In other words, she only had twenty pounds to lose. If she lost the twenty pounds, then she was to consider herself a success without regard to any further losses. This was very motivating for Mrs. Z., and it was extremely gratifying for her when she achieved her first weight loss goal of twenty pounds.

I would say that you should set subgoals of no more than

ten to twenty pound losses if you are very overweight. If you are only fifteen or twenty pounds overweight, then your subgoals should involve losses of only five pounds. When making out your weight loss graph and drawing in the predicted loss line, establish your subgoal. Try to think only of your subgoal. Do not think beyond it if at all possible. If you are very overweight, and think in terms of an eighty or ninety pound weight loss, you will inevitably find yourself becoming discouraged.

Strategies such as this one of setting subgoals may seem shallow and superficial compared to psychoanalytic principles. Analyzing your unconscious motives and understanding your ego defense mechanisms seems to be much more profound. However, I assure you that the goal-gradient hypothesis is just as "deep" a psychological principle as any psychoanalytic principle. It is a valid principle of motivation that applies to behavior on many levels. It is therefore by definition profound. Take advantage of your knowledge of the goal-gradient hypothesis as a weight reduction strategy. *Do* set subgoals for yourself.

HOW TO USE WORK INHIBITION

Another psychological principle that was formulated by Clark L. Hull was the principle of *work inhibition*. The principle is simply this: Whenever we do *anything* there is some work involved. As the work accumulates, an inhibition builds up which motivates us to stop the activity. This is true for *all* activities.

For example, let's say that you are playing Ping-Pong with some friends. The first game is very enjoyable. The second game is also enjoyable. But is the seventh or eighth game enjoyable? Do we not say now that you are getting tired of

Ping-Pong? Is it just a simple matter of getting tired? No, because it is quite possible that you might now enjoy swimming or playing pool. You are not necessarily *fatigued all over*. The key thing here is that you are *tired of* something. This is the key concept in work inhibition. It is the principle of being *tired of* as opposed to the principle of simply *being tired*.

Of course, work inhibition dissipates spontaneously. So after a rest from a particular activity, you may feel like engaging in that activity again. However, according to Hull, whenever there is work inhibition there is the build-up of something else he calls *conditioned inhibition*. Conditioned inhibition is a permanent decrease in the desire to respond to the situation. For example, if someone were to force you to play ten games of Ping-Pong a day, you would find that after a time you might actually come to hate playing Ping-Pong.

How can we apply these principles creatively to dieting? There are several ways. The key thing here is this: *Make the act of eating involve more work than it has in the past.* For example, you could eat all foods on your diet that require quite a bit of chewing. Puddings, malts, doughnuts, and gelatin desserts—these kinds of foods involve little or no chewing. They slip easily from the mouth to the stomach. One of the things you can do to build up work inhibition which in turn will make you want to cease your eating activity is to eat foods—as I said above—that require chewing. For example, if you feel you must have a snack something like beef jerky obviously requires quite a bit of chewing. Unfortunately, most of our snacks require very little chewing. Candy bars, cookies, etc., can all be swallowed with almost no effort. Our food in general is too refined and too processed. So do your best to eat foods that have had a minimum of refinement and processing and you will have to do more chewing. More chewing will lead to a build-up of work inhibition which in turn will help you resist your impulse to continue eating.

One of the things you could do to build up work inhibition is to chew some sugar-free gum for fifteen or twenty minutes just prior to a meal. You will find that your jaws will be somewhat fatigued and you will have received quite a bit of oral gratification. This will make it easier for you to eat less during the meal.

Another thing that some of my clients have found helpful is to consciously and deliberately decide to chew every mouthful of food a certain number of times. For example, one woman decided that she would chew every mouthful of food 20 times. This was of course healthful because the food was thoroughly masticated. But perhaps even more important, she found that it took her "forever" to finish a meal. She was literally tired of eating when her meal was only half consumed. She found that under these conditions she lost all desire for second helpings. She also began to take smaller helpings because she did in fact become tired of eating.

Another way that you can make the act of eating require more work is the simple strategy of putting down your fork and actually *releasing it* between every bite of food. The activity obviously greatly increases the amount of work inhibition that builds up during the meal. It also has the obvious beneficial side effect of making you more conscious of your behavior. When you actually release your fork and set it down you become more aware of the food in your mouth and more aware of your chewing. You will find these strategies very helpful at a social gathering where almost everyone else appears to be happily gobbling their food thinking of second helpings while they are eating their first helpings. Setting your fork down between every bite and counting to ten or twenty with every mouthful of food will give you a certain feeling of distance from the others. You will probably get a feeling that they look to you like happy pigs at an eating trough. Many clients report that a sort of feeling of disdain enters into their perception of the situation. And they feel repulsed by the thought of gobbling up food beyond their immediate needs. You might wonder if others at the social gathering will not notice the fact that you are putting your fork down and taking so long to eat. I assure you that I have found it beneficial to utilize this strategy many times at social gatherings and *no one* notices what I am doing. Even if someone does notice it, so what? Is there anything wrong with eating slowly and thoroughly chewing your food?

A variant on the work inhibition approach is to make it more difficult for yourself to obtain food. Remember Premack's principle of prepotent motivation? If you require yourself to perform a low-probability response in order to execute a high-probability response, the low-probability response will go up and the high-probability response will come down. Concretely, you could utilize this principle as follows: Let's say that you are alone at home, and you want a snack. This is compulsive because you realize you don't need the snack and you are going off your diet. You could introduce something that requires quite a bit of work—a low probability response in Premack's terms—such as running in place to the count of 50 or 100 prior to having the snack. This will give you some needed exercise if you do it. And if you do do it, and still want the snack, then go ahead and have it without guilt. Don't try to use willpower to resist the snack. The only willpower you want to use is the willpower to say to yourself, "If I am to have the snack, I must pay the price by running in place to the count of 100." You will find that if you systematically apply this, you will be running in place more often and getting some needed exercise, and you will also find that often your desire for the snack is gone after paying the price. The work inhibition that builds up during the running period and the conditioned inhibition that builds up over days and weeks becomes associated with having snacks, and you will find that there is a general lowering of your desire to have snacks—probably because of your resistance to doing the work required to have a snack.

I had one client, a young lady of twenty-three, who used this strategy of exercising prior to having a snack. Hearing this discussed in one of my psychology of weight control classes, she decided she would vary my suggestion by running around the block if she was to have a snack. She reported beneficial results in glowing terms. She was jogging and getting some needed exercise, and at the same time she was doing less snacking.

STIMULUS SUBSTITUTION

One of the oldest and most well-known psychological principles for weight control is one we can call *stimulus substitution*. It is perhaps so obvious that one almost hesitates to mention it, feeling that only familiar territory is being covered. Nevertheless, the principle is so basic that attention should be brought to it.

The principle of stimulus substitution was formulated aptly by an old cigarette commercial in the 1930s: "Reach for a Lucky instead of a sweet." Here in this ad we see the principle of stimulus substitution at work. The stimulus to which a person has been conditioned is candy. When he craves something in his mouth he has developed a habit of eating candy. The ad suggests that he might not be able to do away with his craving to put something into his mouth, but that perhaps he can satisfy his craving with a cigarette instead of candy. Perhaps all of this is rather obvious, but nevertheless, more than one overweight person has found it possible to restrict food intake by taking up or continuing with a cigarette-smoking habit. I am not, of course, making a recommendation that you become a smoker if you are not one now. I merely cited the smoking example as a clear and easily grasped illustration of the principle of stimulus substitution in action.

I think the point is that much overeating is due to an abnormal oral craving in which it is necessary to put *something* in the mouth. And sometimes almost anything will do.

I have hit upon coffee drinking as a substitute oral activity for eating. Many days I drink eight to ten cups of coffee. I realize that this is a most reprehensible activity, that coffee is filled with caffeine and acid. But don't you think that this is less damaging to one's health than being seventy pounds overweight, as I once was? Actually, I have recently hit on the idea of drinking either decaffeinated or acid-free coffee. I find either of these substitutes as satisfying as ordinary coffee. Because I clearly see that what I want is not coffee *per se* but something in my mouth.

One of my clients told me that the previous day she had been overwhelmed with a tremendous compulsion to eat. As much as she wanted to eat, she didn't want to become fat again. (She had recently lost sixty pounds, and was now a normal weight.) So instead, in a desperate effort to control her compulsion to eat, she ate a total of eight large carrots in one evening. She was able to avoid eating the cake, cookies, and other sweets in the house by this strategy.

She complained to me about having to do this. She felt that there was something wrong with having to stuff eight large carrots into her mouth in a single evening in order to control her compulsion.

I certainly agree that we want to work on getting rid of our compulsions. The self-analysis of your unconscious motives and ego defenses is a step in this direction. But sometimes, in spite of our best efforts at self-analysis and self-understanding, compulsions have a way of returning. At these times we need a strategy—a psychological "life preserver"—that will give us a way to deal with the compulsion in a practical manner. So I complimented my client on eating the eight carrots instead of berating her for having the compulsion. She had fought a battle and she had won!

In spite of self-analysis and understanding our deeper motivational structure, persons who have had great oral cravings in the past will find from time to time these cravings returning. At these critical moments do not "throw in the towel." Instead, give into the oral craving if you must. But substitute something that won't make you fat: chewing gum, sugar-free soft drinks, beef jerky, cottage cheese, carrots, celery, etc.

As I said before, the principle of stimulus substitution is fairly obvious. But it is also very important. It can be a way out when you are losing self-control. Be sure to remember it and use it.

HABITANALYSIS

The overall habit of eating incorrectly can be analyzed into a set of smaller habits. It can be very valuable to make this analysis. This is much like looking at a drop of water through a microscope. All sorts of things are seen that were invisible before. What we might call *habitanalysis* does this to your overall eating behavior. When you see your bad eating habits revealed on a one-by-one basis it makes it much easier to deal with them. The first step in habitanalysis is to make a list of your most undesirable eating habits and the conditions that trigger these habits. Here is the list of one client, Jane X.:

STIMULUS CONDITION	HABIT PATTERN
1. Friday night	Harry and I go out for Mexican food. I eat a taco, enchilada, beans, rice, and take ice cream for dessert. I eat it all.
2. Morning coffee break	Almost always take a doughnut, Danish, or other sweet. (I work in a bank.)
3. Saturday afternoon alone at home without Harry and the kids.	I raid the refrigerator looking for anything in sight. Usually want a big sandwich.
4. Driving home from work at 4:30 P.M.	Almost always stop for a hamburger and fries even though we'll eat dinner about 7 P.M.
5. Birthdays of relatives	Usually take a large piece of cake and a double scoop of ice cream.
6. Lunch with the girls at work.	Usually take dessert—pie, ice cream, etc. Also, eat two slices of bread with my meal.
7. Dinner at home.	Usually take seconds of starchy foods—rice, potatoes, spaghetti, barley, etc.
8. Breakfast.	I usually skip breakfast. I try to get by on two cups of black coffee. I know I should have something.
9. Passing candy machine in the hall at work.	Can seldom pass it more than three times in a row without getting a candy bar.
10. Shopping at a particular discount store. They have an ice cream counter.	Almost always break down and can't resist the ice cream. Usually get a double dip.

Jane handed her list to me with this comment: "Here's my list of bad eating habits. Until I did this, I don't think I realized just how bad my eating habits are. Looking over the list it's a wonder to me that I'm not fatter than I am. I used to think 'why am I so fat?' There's not much of a mystery to it. It's my eating habits."

The first step in the habitanalysis is simply to list the most important bad eating habits and the stimulus conditions that evoke the habits. The second step is to *rank* the habits according to strength. In Jane's case I suggested that she copy her list onto a set of 3 x 5 index cards, using one card for each habit. On the front of the card I asked her to place the stimulus condition and the habit pattern. On the back of each card she was to jot down any habit-breaking ideas she or I could generate together. The index cards make it easy to rank the habits. The strongest habit is placed at the *bottom* of the pile, and the weakest habit is at the *top*. The reason for doing this is that we want to try to eliminate the habits *in reverse order*. One works on the weakest habits first. The idea is that it is much easier to eliminate or modify a weak habit than a strong habit. But what about the strong habits? Fortunately, there is something in conditioning theory called the *generalization of extinction*. What this means in practical terms is that getting rid of one bad habit will have a weakening effect on other bad habits. Think of the ranked habits as a ladder. As you move from the weakest toward the strongest habits, the strongest habits have been losing strength. When you start to work on the strongest habits you will find that they are now no stronger than the first habits you worked on. At this moment you may find this a little hard to believe, but it really works this way. It is usually unrealistic and impractical to think you can eliminate all of your bad habits in one day. Yet this is what most overweight people want to do. They want to move from a set of bad eating habits to a Spartan regimen in one day.

How do you eliminate or modify incorrect eating habits? Many methods have been suggested in this book. I would suggest that you make your set of index cards with the stimulus conditions and habit patterns on the front. Then leaf through the book looking for ideas that pertain to each habit. Jot the ideas down on the back of each card. Then pick out no more than two or three of the weakest habits and try to work on them.

In order to be as concrete as possible about this I am going to present the information on Jane's cards. The original list you saw was just jotted down by Jane at random. The following list is in order of habit strength. I am using Roman numerals in order to indicate the difference.

RANK

I. *Front of card.* Breakfast. I usually skip breakfast. I try to get by on two cups of black coffee.

Back of card. I think this should be the easiest habit to break. I want to eat in the morning. I only skip breakfast because I want to lose weight. Maybe if I have a piece of plain toast without butter or jelly and a glass of skim milk for breakfast I won't need the sweets at coffee break.

II. *Front of card.* Morning coffee break. Almost always take a doughnut, Danish, or other sweet.

Back of card. I think if I have the glass of skim milk for breakfast that the protein in the milk combined with the sugar from the digested starch in the toast should keep my blood sugar level high enough that I can resist the doughnut or Danish. If this doesn't work, I'll try stimulus substitution. I'll have a scoop of cottage cheese instead of a sweet. If that doesn't work, I won't go on break with the girls. I'll stay at my desk and catch up with my work.

III. *Front of card.* Passing candy machine in the hall at work. Can seldom pass it more than three tin... in a row without getting a candy bar.

Back of card. I really don't think much about the candy until I see the machine. I pass it because I go to the rest room that way or I want water. I can keep a thermos of water at my desk. This will cut down on the number of times I see the machine. Also, I can go to the rest room the long way; go outside of the building and walk around it to the other entrance. The walk will do me good and I won't see the candy machine. I think these ideas will work.

At this point in Jane's habitanalysis we stopped trying to generate habit-breaking ideas. It was agreed that Jane would work on the three weakest habits first. If we eliminated these, then we would proceed to the other seven habits. Within two weeks Jane felt that she had gained sufficient control over the three weakest habits that she could move on to the stronger habits.

Here is the information on three more cards:

IV. *Front of card.* Dinner at home: usually take seconds of starchy foods—rice, potatoes, spaghetti, barley, etc.

Back of card. Think I'll try work inhibition on this problem. I am going to deliberately take only one

small helping of starchy food with dinner. Whenever I take a bit of, say, mashed potatoes, I'll take
only a small bite. I'll release my fork—actually put
it down. And I'll count to twenty before I swallow
the bite of mashed potato. This should take the
fun out of it and make me bored with eating
starches. It will take me "forever" to eat a helping
of starchy food, and I won't go for a second
helping.

V. *Front of card.* Driving home from work at 4:30
P.M. Almost always stop for a hamburger and fries
even though we'll eat dinner about 7 P.M.

Back of card. Time to use Premack's principle. I'm
working on an oil painting and taking a painting
class. This is my hobby and main outlet. If I can
pass up the hamburger and fries, I can work on the
oil painting in the evenings. If I don't pass them
up, I can't work on the painting.

VI. *Front of card.* Birthdays of relatives: usually
take a large piece of cake and a double scoop of ice
cream.

Back of card. Am going to ask for a small piece of
cake and no ice cream at all. Then I will eat only
the cake part and leave the frosting which is the
most fattening part. Eliminating the ice cream,
taking a smaller helping, and not eating the frosting
should cut the calories from seven or eight hundred
to about one hundred fifty. I won't be having
many more calories than a glass of milk. And I'll
still be participating in the festivities.

Jane worked on modifying and eliminating the three habits
listed above for about one month. It was now six weeks since

the beginning of her habitanalysis, and she had lost a total of fourteen pounds as a direct result of the improvement in her eating habits. She was eating less starch and sugar and taking in more protein and green vegetables. And informal analysis suggested that she had gone from a diet that was almost fifty per cent sugar and starch to a diet that was twenty-five per cent sugar and starch.

We decided to break down the last four habits into sets of two:

> **VII.** *Front of card.* Shopping at a particular discount store. They have an ice cream counter. Almost always break down and can't resist the ice cream. Usually get a double dip.
>
> *Back of card.* I feel sorry for myself. I hate to go shopping at that store. I think I deserve a treat as I leave. Possibilities: Don't shop there until I lose weight even if it costs me money. Try stimulus substitution. Carry gum in my purse and pop some into my mouth as I check out. When I pass the ice cream I'll be chewing gum and my mouth will be busy with something else. I like iced tea. Have that as a treat instead of ice cream. No sugar of course.
>
> **VIII.** *Front of card.* Lunch with the girls at work. Usually take dessert—pie, ice cream, etc. Also, eat two slices of bread with my meal.
>
> *Back of card.* One reason I go for dessert is because I eat too fast. I'm done eating and the other girls are still working on their meals. This makes me feel deprived, and I get up and go get a dessert. I'm going to work on slowing down. Best idea I know of, at least it's been working well for me, is putting

my fork down between bites and actually *counting* to twenty before proceeding. If I can space out my meal so I still have some food when everybody is done, I think I can resist the dessert.

Jane worked on these two habits for three weeks before proceeding to work on the last two habits. Originally, these last two habits had seemed formidable and almost impossible to break to her. But after succeeding with eight other habits, she approached them with a certain degree of confidence.

IX. *Front of card.* Saturday afternoon alone at home without Harry and the kids. I raid the refrigerator looking for anything in sight. Usually want a big sandwich.

Back of card. I think this would have been impossible to eliminate or modify a few weeks ago. But now I've got a few ideas that should work. If the going gets too rough, I think I'll just get in the car and go for a ride. I'm going to stop feeling so guilty about getting the housework done on Saturday. I work at the bunk all week. I'm going to keep the refrigerator stocked with guilt-free snacks: dill pickles, beef jerky, and low-calorie soda. I'll satisfy my mouth hunger this way. I'm *not* going to eat the foods that make me fat.

X. *Front of card.* Friday night. Harry and I go out for Mexican food. I eat a taco, enchilada, beans, rice, and take ice cream for dessert. I eat it all.

Back of card. When I started all this I never thought I'd break this habit. But I guess the generalization of extinction is working. Because Harry and I have already skipped going twice since I

started working on my other habits. Since I've lost
some weight my desire for rich foods has declined.
I think I'll handle this one by going for Mexican
food only once a month instead of every week.
Also, I'm going to just leave some of the beans and
rice on the plate.

Jane found it very easy to work on the last two habits.
Indeed, they turned out to be the easiest to eliminate of all
ten when she at last got to working on them. Success begets
success, and her previous work on her other habits paid off
across the board. In approximately two months Jane had
mastered her worst eating habits. She had lost eighteen
pounds.

I cannot stress too strongly the importance of actually
making a habitanalysis on paper. It brings order to chaos, and
it gives you a systematic approach to your eating problems.
The "shotgun" approach is worthless. You can't eliminate all
of your bad eating habits in one day. And you have got to
analyze the strategies you intend to use to deal with your
habits. The method suggested in this section gives you a
practical way of doing this.

The ideas offered in this chapter on creative weight control
are among the most powerful ideas offered in this book.
They are based on a large and important subfield of scientific
psychology called *learning theory*. Of course, nothing works
unless you actually do it. So it's up to you. Give the ideas in
this chapter a chance. Apply them to yourself and start losing
weight.

Chapter 7

Between Husband and Wife

There is no lament more commonly heard by marriage counselors than this one: "We can't communicate!" More often than not it is the wife who first goes to a marriage counselor. (This is a fact. Women are much more willing to seek professional help when a marriage is in trouble.) Mrs. Betty J.'s opening remarks are typical: "I don't know what's wrong with Harry and me. We just don't seem to be able to communicate any more. I ask him to do even a simple thing like throw out the garbage and he has a fit. We can't discuss politics, religion, or the children without getting into an argument. It's just hopeless. He seems so cold and distant now—nothing like when we dated."

Betty's marriage is not unusual. The poor quality of communication between her and her husband has reduced their once loving relationship to a caricature of a relationship.

We might ask ourselves what are the goals of marriage? The answers that tend to come to mind are: to raise children, to have a satisfying sexual relationship, to acquire financial security, and to provide companionship. Let's take the last idea—*to provide companionship*. This is a more powerful concept than we might realize. A really good marriage provides companionship. That is to say that a really good marriage reduces our feelings of isolation and loneliness in this world. A happily married person is not alienated. He (or she) feels that he belongs in this world. If you are happily married, this helps you feel you have status and an identity. And this state of affairs arises from the fact that at least one other human being in this world really knows you and cares about you. In his book *Games People Play* Eric Berne called this happy state of affairs *intimacy*. And it should be the goal of any personal relationship (husband, wife, parent and child, close friends, etc.) where the relationship is not a means to an end.

At this point we might distinguish between *intrinsic* relationships and *extrinsic* relationships. An intrinsic relationship is one where the returns should come from the relationship itself. As noted above, the relationship is not a means to an end. These relationships must involve genuine caring and real concern for the other person, otherwise they are "dead." They are dull, lifeless affairs in which the other person has become a thing instead of a human being. The philosopher Martin Buber spoke of loving relationships as I-thou relationships as opposed to I-it relationships. His feeling was that wherever possible we should cultivate with other members of the human race an I-thou relationship. It is only in this way that we can overcome our feeling of isolation and loneliness.

An extrinsic relationship is one in which we see the relationship as a means to an end. To illustrate, let's say that a student is taking a psychology class from me. He sees me only as a way of getting three college units and a grade. He does everything I ask—and he gets his units and his grade. But he is bored by the class, never asks an interesting question, never participates in a discussion, never engages me in conversation outside of the class. We have come nowhere near having an I-thou relationship. He has *used* me. He has reduced me to a thing. I could just as well have been a programmed robot teaching him for all he cared.

The same failing may emanate from the teacher. His students bore him. He doesn't care to learn their names or anything about them. If they approach him outside of class, he cringes and doesn't want to get involved. We've all known teachers like this. They shouldn't be teaching. They are using their students as a means to an end: to get a paycheck. They have reduced their students to things by their attitudes.

Let's face facts. It is not always possible to establish an I-thou relationship with everyone you meet. For example, you can't always do it with your boss. The paycheck you get from him may be much more important to you than any other aspect of your relationship. However, even in this relationship it might be possible to be more open and honest. Many employees swallow all kinds of "guff" because they think they have to take it. They come to despise their employers and hate their jobs. In fact the employer might be a lot more approachable than the employee thinks. But the employee cannot take risks because of fear.

But let's return to the relationship between husband and wife. Certainly in this relationship—if nowhere else—we should strive for the goal of psychological and emotional intimacy. Your relationship with your spouse should be an I-thou relationship. Your wife or husband is not a thing to be manipulated. Unfortunately, too many marriages end up "dead." They are the burned-out hulks of once flaming love affairs.

What does all of this have to do with you and overeating? Just this: The state of your marriage has a great deal to do with problems that plague the overweight person. Eating between meals, a compulsion to overeat, food binging, and raiding the refrigerator in the middle of the night can all be reactions to negative feelings arising from a poor marriage relationship.

COMMUNICATION PROBLEMS

Some years ago an expert in semantics and communication named Wendell Johnson wrote a book called *People in Quandaries*. In this book he spoke of something called the I-F-D syndrome. I-F-D stands for idealization, frustration, and despair. Johnson's point was this: Very often in life we enter situations and relationships with happy anticipation, simplifying and denying reality because of our strong wish for the world to fit our needs. This is the *idealization* stage. Seldom does reality match our expectations. And this leads to a second stage, *frustration*. The first reaction to frustration is anger. But if frustration is long-standing, anger deteriorates into depression.

The I-F-D syndrome can be applied to many things in life. But let's see how it works applied to marriage. As I write I am thinking of a young married woman, Mrs. Marie C. Marie was engaged for one year prior to her marriage. During this period she and her mother planned a beautiful wedding, and Marie got married in a cloud of glory. She looked and felt like a fairy princess on her wedding day. During the period of her engagement her fiance, Tom, took her to good restaurants and live theatre frequently. She saw little faults in Tom—but she brushed them aside. The fact that he was given to sulky moods, smoked heavily, was often glued to the television set during baseball games, and seemed to drink too much beer were minor irritations. We have here a restatement of the old saying, "Love is blind." There is a great deal of wisdom in that short phrase. Our perception distorts reality according to our needs. And so Marie didn't see Tom when she looked at Tom. She saw an image—she saw what she wanted to see. (Mental health workers call this *autistic thinking*. Mental patients are dominated by their needs. They see and hear what they want to hear. But mental patients aren't the only ones who engage in autistic thinking. We all do it to a certain extent.) So when Marie thought of what it would be like to be married, she did not have mental pictures that conformed to what the reality of marriage would be. She naively pictured herself in a lovely new tract home with modern furnishings. She gave no consideration to how she and Tom would attain this status.

It is obvious that Marie had built herself up for a fall. When she and Tom moved into a small apartment without air conditioning she loved it at first. It all seemed like a dream come true. Her own apartment where she and Tom could entertain her friends! But in a few years Marie was a very disillusioned young lady. She had one child, she was pregnant with another one, she hated to do diapers, and she and Tom could not afford a diaper service. Tom made a reasonable income at a fair job, but it did not provide a standard of living that matched Marie's picture of how they should be living. They had moved into a new tract home—but there was still no air conditioning. And Southern California summers are hot! She had only a few pieces of good furniture, and there was certainly no sense of integration or theme to the decorations in the home.

Something had gone wrong. Marie couldn't put her finger on it. She still loved Tom—or thought she did. And divorce was seldom on her mind. Nevertheless, his interest in television sports events and his incessant beer drinking were now clear irritants. Sometimes she felt like screaming at him, "Put down that beer can and do some work around here! Can't you see the lawns need mowing!" She seldom "blew her top." Once in a while she did. But Tom had a tendency to laugh it off with a joke and open another can of beer. He was difficult to engage in a quarrel.

The disenchantment that Marie felt with her marriage was equivalent to Wendell Johnson's second stage, *frustration*. She was frustrated and she knew it. She often asked herself questions such as: Why didn't I wait a little longer to get married? Why didn't I go to college? Is it too late now? What would it be like to be married to someone else? But asking these questions made her only more frustrated.

Anger and depression were the inevitable result. She sank apathetically into the third stage of the I-F-D syndrome. A kind of permanent gray depression settled over her life. She went on day by day in a mode of conscious noncaring. Life was just a chore to be gotten through. She developed a habit of eating when she felt lonely, eating when she felt tired, and eating when she felt unhappy. And she felt lonely, tired, and unhappy often. So she ate often. And she got fat. By the time she was married five years she was fifty pounds overweight. She had gained ten pounds for every year of marriage. The once trim young girl looked like a middle-aged woman at the age of twenty-five.

Did Marie and Tom have communication problems? They certainly did. And when did their troubles start? I think we can fairly say that the seeds of their problems were planted during the engagement period. Neither Marie nor Tom used the engagement period constructively. They did not discuss their future in a realistic way. Tom tried to present himself as a sophisticated man-about-town. Marie bought the image because she wanted to. And they were both hurt as a result.

In the case of Marie and Tom we have an illustration of a communication problem that existed from the early stages of their relationship. They thought they communicated because they chattered happily about things they saw and did—but this is not communication. It is just what I have called in the previous sentence—chatter. I have said this not to downgrade the importance of small talk; but it should be secondary to a sounder and more fundamental understanding between people.

If I had a word of advice for engaged couples, it would be to exchange views on serious topics before you get married. Talk about politics, sex, religion, child rearing, and money before you take your vows. An exchange of views on an honest basis may reduce your expectations and your realization. There are people who say it is wrong to reduce idealization, that it is very beautiful to see people looking at the world through rose-colored glasses. I disagree. It is easier to come off a cloud before marriage than after marriage. The person who enters marriage with a realistic outlook is less likely to experience frustration, anger, and depression after marriage.

None of this may apply to you. You're already married. And it's too late for you to do anything about the engagement period. Let's make the assumption that in your marriage communication is far from what you want it to be. What can you do to improve matters? Hopefully, this chapter will give you a few insights and some practical ideas.

GAMES FAT PEOPLE PLAY

In accordance with Eric Berne's *Games People Play*, a "game" may be defined as a set of stereotyped transactions in which the players have ulterior motives. In order to have a game there must be at least two players: an antagonist and a protagonist. What this means applied to marriage is that many exchanges between husband and wife tend to become routine and all too predictable. People manipulate each other and they don't even know why they are doing it on a conscious level. People are literally "players," "playing games" without knowing it. The ulterior goal of many marriage games is *aggression:* to hurt the marital partner. The value in describing games is that the description makes us more aware of our own behavior, and in consequence potentially more objective. There is then some hope of breaking the game and moving toward *intimacy* or real communication. Let's describe a few of the games fat people and their spouses play.

JACK SPRAT'S WIFE

We have all heard the nursery rhyme:

> Jack Sprat could eat no fat
> His wife could eat no lean
> And so between the two of them
> They licked the platter clean

This familiar work from Mother Goose reveals that *Jack Sprat's Wife* is a game that has been played for many years. I am calling it a game because it is not at all unusual to see a marriage in which one partner is obese and the other partner is underweight. It is a very common pattern. The "Jack Sprat" character can be either the wife or the husband. The point is that one of the partners overeats and the other partner undereats. The fatter the fat partner gets, the thinner the thin partner gets. I know a couple where one's weight gain is almost always counterbalanced by the other member's weight loss. The wife has recently gained twenty pounds. The husband has recently lost twenty pounds and says, "I can't gain it back no matter how hard I try."

What is going on here, and why is it a game? The really hard player, the antagonist, in this game is the thin person. He loses weight and remains thin because unconsciously it makes him feel *superior* to the wife. Jack Sprat is saying on a nonverbal level, "See how superior I am to you. See how much self-control and character I have compared to you."

This superior attitude makes the overweight person all the more frustrated and prone to overeat. Why does Jack Sprat's wife play? What is she getting out of the game? At first glance, it would appear she gets nothing. It is absurd to let another person feel superior at your expense. That is what rational thinking tells us. But the game—all of the games—operate at a more or less unconscious irrational level. Jack Sprat's wife plays because of a masochistic need to feel more worthless than she already feels. In a word she has a need for *self-abasement.*

A need for self-abasement usually arises from long-standing feelings of guilt. These feelings of guilt may arise from real transgressions in the past. For example, I knew a Jack Sprat's wife who had had an abortion prior to her marriage. She had been sexually intimate with a young man who was later jailed for a felony. Subsequently, she married an "upstanding" citizen, concealing the fact of the abortion. But she felt undeserving of her status. She had never worked through her feelings of guilt for the abortion.

Chronic feelings of guilt may also arise from what might be called "thought-crimes." Jack Sprat's wife feels unworthy not because of what she does, but because of what she thinks. I remember one obese woman who dreamed off and on for five years of having a sexual affair with her brother-in-law. She never actually *did* anything with her brother-in-law.

But she masturbated at least once a week enjoying vivid sexual fantasies with her brother-in-law. These sexual fantasies were much more exciting to her than actual sex relations with her husband. She looked forward to masturbating and fantasizing much more than she looked forward to overt sexual relations with her spouse.

This particular woman was a client, and fortunately her feelings of guilt were greatly reduced by talking them through in psychotherapy. She began to lose weight immediately.

If you are playing the part of Jack Sprat's wife, ask yourself why you put up with the game. Do you see any real or imagined events in your life that are making you feel guilty? The odds are you have already paid enough. Try to break the pattern of the game by asking yourself what you are getting out of it. Self-punishment is a futile activity. A famous rabbi once asked, "Are you for yourself or against yourself?" This great question implies a great deal. Are you on a positive road of self-improvement? Or are you punishing yourself and destroying yourself? If you are doing the latter, then you are your own worst enemy. Try to think these questions through and put an end to self-destructive behavior. Stop playing the part of Jack Sprat's wife. In the end you are only hurting yourself. You are helping no one.

WATCHED DOG

The two players in this game are the *watchdog* and the *watched dog*. The watched dog is the overweight person. The husband or the wife can play either part depending on who is a normal weight and who is overweight. Sometimes an overweight couple will play both parts simultaneously. But let's simplify and stick to the situation in which only one partner is overweight.

The ulterior or unconscious motive operating in *watched dog* for the one playing the part of watchdog is the need to control others. This individual may have what psychologists call an *authoritarian personality*. An authoritarian personality makes a good dictator. He cannot tolerate uncertainty. The world must be ordered and predictable. If the wife is a watchdog, she will also have a tendency to be an extremely neat and orderly housekeeper. She will nag her husband to clean his feet outside very carefully before entering the house. The children will be scolded often because they are unkempt. Everything in the house will stand at attention—from the furniture to the pictures. If the husband is a watchdog, he will also have a tendency to be preoccupied with neatness and order. His garage will have a place for every tool, his suits will always be pressed and ready to wear, his car will be polished every week, and so forth. I hope you realize that I am not speaking out against neatness and cleanliness—but anything can be overdone.

The motive operating in the watched dog is a desire for freedom. He feels overcontrolled. Overeating is a way of being temporarily free of the power of the watchdog. The importance of the concept of freedom in compulsive eating can hardly be overemphasized. A compulsive eater seems to be anything but free. However, freedom is a word that is often difficult to construe properly. Freedom can mean an acting out of one's own impulses as a way of fighting off the outer control of another personality. A client—a watched dog—told me the following story, "My wife sent me on a rush errand to the grocery story. It was almost an order. So I'm an agreeable guy. I didn't argue. But I resented the high-handed way she practically ordered me to go. I remember acting okay about it—cheerful, on the outside. But inside I was angry. So on the way to the store I had this pleasant thought, 'I'll get an ice cream cone and eat it as I drive home. Alice will never know about it.' Then I got an insight that I really think is an important one. I saw that my planned action of buying an ice cream cone was my attempt to carve out a tiny area of freedom in my 'unfree' act of going to the grocery store. When I got this insight I realized what a pathetic thing it was. Here I am—obese—and I think I'm striking a blow for freedom by my act of sneaking an ice cream cone. When I got to the grocery store and saw the ice cream counter I said to myself, 'You think you're being free by buying that ice cream cone behind your wife's back. But that's not freedom—that's compulsion!' I told myself I should have both the courage to eat in front of Alice when I want to, and also the courage to express my resentment at her ordering me about."

Here is another example of how a watched dog overeats as a way of feeling free of the power of the watchdog. A wife I know keeps herself in a constant state of agitation over her husband's "eating problem." She is an example of the worst kind of watchdog. At a dinner party she will say, "I'll fix Harry's plate. You know he's not to have too many carbohydrates." Or, "No thank you. Harry doesn't want any bread. You know he's trying to reduce." You wouldn't think that Harry would stand still for this. But he just sits there and smiles—seeming to go along with his wife. And yet every year Harry gets fatter and fatter. His wife is only making the problem worse. She doesn't see the sneak eating Harry does. Harry has taken to stopping in a topless bar two or three afternoons a week when he can get off work a half-hour early. His wife is unaware of this small escapade on Harry's part. It is a tiny area of personal freedom for him. He flirts with the topless dancers, drinks three or four beers (loaded with carbohydrates) and munches large handfuls of nuts and pretzels (also loaded with carbohydrates). He goes home fatter and happier. How can his wife's being a watchdog possibly be of any help to him? Harry can't be motivated by treating him like a wayward child. You can't pump motivation into a human being the same way you pump air into a balloon. The generalization holds right across the board: A watchdog makes a watched dog. And a watched dog wants to be free.

If you are the one who is the watched dog, you should try to remember the words of the client quoted earlier in this section: "I saw that my planned action of buying an ice cream cone was my attempt to carve out a tiny area of freedom in my 'unfree' act of going to the store. When I got this insight I realized what a pathetic thing it was. Here I am—obese—and I think I'm striking a blow for freedom by my act of sneaking an ice cream cone." This client has hit the nail right on the head. He has analyzed his reactions, and as a consequence has attained a measure of self-control.

MOMMY'S LITTLE BOY

The game of *Mommy's Little Boy* obviously requires a mommy and a little boy. In this game the mommy stuffs the little boy with food and makes him fat. The wife who is playing the part of a mommy has a need to prove to herself that she loves her husband. This is the ulterior motive operating within her. She may have a great deal of resentment toward her husband. Acts of "mothering" her husband make her feel better about herself. She tries to prove to herself that her hostile feelings are not there by, what seem to be on the surface, acts of affection: cooking rich foods, baking tempting desserts. But these fattening foods have a double meaning. She can feel she is being loving and affectionate while she is killing her husband. You think this is too harsh? A friend of mine recently commented, "My aunt killed my uncle with her oven." This occurred in spite of the fact that the aunt knew her husband was suffering from malignant hypertension aggravated by obesity. She continued to cook rich foods in the face of special diets prescribed by the family physician. When her husband died suddenly of a heart attack she was grief-stricken for weeks. One wonders how grief-stricken she was at the deepest levels of her personality.

The need operating in the one playing the part of the little boy is a need to comply. The husband wishes to "please" mommy. He can't say no. Perhaps down deep he feels unloved by his wife. These feelings may be complicated by a feeling that his real mother doesn't love him. Without realizing it, he has transferred his feelings from his real mother to his wife. He still wants his mother's approval. And so he thinks he can gain the love of both his mother and his wife by eating his wife's food.

If you are playing the part of the little boy, try to face the problem squarely. You can't gain your wife's love by eating her food. Try to resist overtures to "take just a little piece of pie. I baked it just for you." Resistance will raise your anxiety level and hers. But it is the only way of moving away from the game toward intimacy.

DADDY'S LITTLE GIRL

The game of *Daddy's Little Girl* is almost the same as the game of *Mommy's Little Boy*. The roles have been reversed. The unconscious motives operating are the same ones. The daddy is trying to prove to himself that he loves his wife. The little girl has a need to comply in order to maintain her husband's love.

A husband playing the part of daddy may bring home boxes of candy for his wife from time to time even though it is obvious she is obese and doesn't need the food. Candy is his favorite gift to her on her birthday, Valentine's Day, Christmas, Easter, and their wedding anniversary. Of course the daddy rationalizes that "he doesn't know what else to buy." But this is a thin rationalization. He could just as well settle on the unimaginative cologne that some men buy as the traditional box of candy. He could bring flowers, a book, or a gift certificate. But he persists in bringing the candy. Food is the symbol of love for this man. If he feeds you, he loves you.

The daddy husband will take his wife out to dinner often. If he can afford it, he will take his wife to better restaurants. He will encourage her to make exceptions, although on the surface he may agree that she should diet and lose weight. How is this possible? By the aid of double-talk: "Why don't you go ahead and have the chocolate eclair tonight, Sally. It really looks delicious there on the dessert tray. I promise you we'll both go on a diet tomorrow. Let's make this one last fling!"

Remember that the little girl has a need to comply. She thinks she will lose her husband's love if she does not do what he asks her to do. She feels she must eat the food he offers or he will feel rejected. So she eats the candy he brings home and eats the food he encourages her to eat when they go out.

If you are caught up in this situation, what can you do? First, look at things realistically. Again, you can't gain love by eating food. You might consider telling your husband that you no longer want candy as a gift. If he persists in bringing it in spite of your reasonable request, you can ask him to return it unopened. I know of one wife who accepted the candy lovingly. When her husband was at work she dropped two or three pieces of candy down the garbage disposal. Everybody was happy. The husband was not confronted. The wife enjoyed throwing the candy away. It was an act of aggression toward her husband. She had come to feel that his bringing her candy was an aggressive act on his part. So she "got back" at him by throwing it away. I'm not sure I recommend what she did. It is obviously more game playing. The couple is certainly not moving toward intimacy when things like this go on. Nevertheless, her behavior helped her reduce. And this is important in and of itself.

YO-YO

You will perhaps recall Mrs. C. who was mentioned briefly in Chapter 3 on the ego defense mechanisms. I stated that I have seen her go from obesity to a normal weight and back again seven times. In the game of *Yo-Yo* the overweight person plays the part of the yo-yo, and the spouse plays the part of string holder. Once again, either part may be played by either partner.

The hard player in this game is the one playing the part of the yo-yo. He or she is always on a compulsive eating jag or on a compulsive dieting jag. Mrs. C., a typical human yo-yo, played the game primarily as a sadistic activity. It was a way of punishing Mr. C. As she lost weight, the poor man dared to hope that maybe this time she would stay normal in her appearance. But just when the treasure was almost in his reach, she would yank it away. The first compliment, the first sign of approval on his part, would be her cue to start her compulsive eating again. We're all familiar with the phrase, "cat and mouse game." The yo-yo game is really a variant of the old cat and mouse game: First you give and then you take. What else did Mrs. C. get out of the game? During her periods of compulsive dieting she felt drunk with power. She felt she was the master of her fate and the captain of her soul. During these periods she was capable of staying on almost any kind of diet. Very restricted diets were her forté. It made her feel noble and self-sacrificing.

Mr. C., the string holder, was a fairly passive player in this game. Nevertheless, he was getting something out of it, and that is why he continued to play. His part might also be called "jerk" or "dummy." He was letting someone manipulate him and make a fool out of him. Why? In his particular case he had a secret feeling that he didn't deserve Mrs. C. It brought tears to his eyes when he thought of her on her wedding day. She was so slim and lovely! Her parents had made him promise to "take good care of our little girl." But Mr. C. had failed twice in business, and felt humiliated before his in-laws. Although Mr. and Mrs. C. did not live in the slums, their modest home was far below the inner standards Mr. C. had set for himself. He felt he deserved to be punished for his failures.

To summarize, Mrs. C. was sadistic in her behavior: Her goal was to punish. Mr. C. was masochistic: His goal was to be punished. They had what psychologists call a sado-masochistic relationship. They met each other's pathological needs.

You may be noting that the dynamics of *Yo-Yo* are very similar to the dynamics of *Jack Sprat's Wife.* Jack Sprat and his wife also have what is basically a sado-masochistic relationship. You will recall that Jack Sprat wanted to feel superior and his wife wanted to abase herself. However, the complexities of games are such that in the case of *Yo-Yo* it is the overweight person who is the sadistic one. In Jack Sprat the thin partner is sadistic. The interplay of unconscious motives in games can lead to such seemingly paradoxical outcomes.

The string holder in the game of *Yo-Yo* is not always as passive as Mr. C. If the string holder has any sadistic tendencies himself, he may be more rejecting toward his wife when she is slim than when she is fat. I know of one husband who makes no sexual advances toward his wife when she is a normal weight. She has to gain weight to gain sex.

STOPPING THE GAMES

It would be possible to present more games. But I think you get the idea. People frequently do play games. Married couples often manipulate each other for obscure reasons. Not all married couples have fallen into the trap of playing games. But game playing is all too common. Games are undesirable and unconstructive because they kill the real humanity between two people. The relationship becomes I-it instead of I-thou. Genuine caring is lost. The potential of human intimacy is destroyed.

So how do you stop a game? You stop a marriage game the way you stop any game. Someone gets bored with the game. Or someone breaks the rules. Or someone just calls a halt and walks away from the game. It takes two people to play the game, and if one person refuses to play, the game is over. This usually results in an *encounter* or a *confrontation* between the couple. Anger is expressed. As a consequence, the couple will either move away from each other toward divorce or separation. Or they will move close together toward intimacy.

One can't make a categorical prediction about what will happen to a couple when one of their games is disrupted. A great deal depends on the basic foundation of their marriage. If it is firm, the disruption of a game will have a long-run beneficial effect. The couple will draw closer together. If the basic foundation of their marriage is weak, the disruption of one or several games may lead to the dissolution of the marriage.

The risks are obviously there. And so it is understandable that people often draw back from encounters and confrontations. I think much of the problem revolves around the fact that people often do not know how to express their real feelings without "shooting the works." They store grievances and hold their tongues for weeks or months at a time. When they risk an encounter it almost always seems to have a depressing effect on the marriage because too much comes out all at once. Anger should be expressed little by little on a daily basis, not in one great storm.

We come back to opening remarks of this chapter. The complaint, "We can't communicate," is a common one. Let's examine some of the ways couples can improve their communication.

COMMUNICATION GUIDELINES

How couples communicate has been studied extensively by psychotherapists and students of semantics. It is not a vague subject. Very definite things can be said about effective communication, and it is a tragedy that more people are not aware of what these things are. Some of the key guidelines to open an effective communication are presented in the remaining pages of this chapter. We are still concerned with weight control. Let's grant that some people are "food-aholics"—that they eat when they are frustrated, bored, or depressed. Let's also grant that many of these negative emotions arise due to poor communication between husband and wife. It is thus clear that an improvement in communication can have two positive values: (1) It can help people stop playing games, and (2) it can help alleviate the problem of overeating.

BE OPEN

Perhaps you recall the poem "A Poison Tree" by William Blake:

> I was angry with my friend:
> I told my wrath, my wrath did end.
> I was angry with my foe:
> I told it not, my wrath did grow.

This is not the whole poem. But the four lines quoted express the central point. Blake wrote the poem in the eighteenth century, but the truth expressed in the poem is universal. If you contain your anger toward your spouse, your anger will grow and poison your relationship. If you express your anger, it will evaporate. Real feelings must be vented. You can't keep them locked up forever. If you do, you will pay with psychosomatic symptoms: muscular tension, headaches, possibly ulcers, and so forth. And don't think that obesity is not a psychosomatic disorder. It is. It is thus a condition that is aggravated by a poor marriage relationship. Clearly, you must be an authentic person. You must "tell your wrath" and it will end.

But how? How can you be open and keep your partner's affection at the same time? There are a number of ways of doing it.

KEEP A COMPLAINT SPECIFIC

One of the most common errors that married people make is that they fail to keep their complaints specific. A husband may issue such complaints as:

"You're a lousy housekeeper."
"You're never going to learn to cook."
"You never want sex."
"You just don't understand my ambitions."
"You're not training the kids right."

A wife may bring forth the following complaints:

"You don't ever get my car repaired."
"You never see what needs to be done in the yard."
"You always want sex at the wrong time."
"You don't play with the children enough."
"All you want to do on weekends is watch television."

The complaints are usually made after the aggravated person has had all she or he can stand. Usually, the aggravated person feels very saintly and righteous. The complaint seems obvious and correct. The complainer often experiences substantial surprise when the other person becomes defensive.

The person who has been criticized usually feels defensive for some very good reasons. First of all, his character has been attacked. A generalization has been made about his personality. Secondly, he can think of many exceptions to the complaint.

You should never issue a complaint in the form of a sweeping generalization. The husband who says, "You're never going to learn to cook," probably means something such as, "You overcooked the roast tonight." This is what he should say. He can say it loudly. He can say it with anger. And he can and should say it every time it happens, assuming it really aggravates him. If it happens every other night, it's probably a good idea to complain every other night. But if, instead, he waits a week and then says, "You're never going to learn to cook," his wife will immediately think of the three times that week that the food was not overcooked. She will feel hurt—and rightly so. His statement was not correct. It was only a partial truth.

The wife who says, "You never see what needs to be done in the yard," probably means something such as, "We're having the family for dinner tomorrow afternoon. I wish you would mow the lawn between now and then." This latter statement is specific and deals with the couple's world at a concrete level. The charge that the husband never sees what needs to be done in the yard is much too abstract. The husband thinks of the last time he mowed the lawn, the Sunday he spent pruning roses, the day he spread fertilizer on his own initiative, and so forth. No wonder he feels wounded by his wife's charge.

So keep your complaints specific. You may still argue. But at least you'll be arguing about something real, not a vague abstraction that you can't point at.

HOW TO AVOID NAME-CALLING AND LABELS

It almost seems too obvious to say in black and white that you should avoid name-calling and labels. Almost everyone knows you shouldn't do it. And yet I know otherwise intelligent people who engage in this activity. One wife I know with a college degree has, from time to time in the past few years, called her husband the following names: meathead, jerk, slob, pig, fool, and fatso. She started the name-calling. But lately he has responded with: lazy, shiftless, nag, bitch, and shrew. They throw the names at each other like bricks when they are arguing. And, like bricks, they hurt.

How can you avoid such nonconstructive activity? The wife told me, "How can I not call him names? He *is* a meathead." If your reaction is about the same as hers, I think you have to remind yourself that a term such as meathead is once again a gross generalization. It is an abstraction about the other person's personality. The old saw, "All generalizations are false including this one," can be applied here. The poor guy can't be a meathead all of the time. Aren't there times when he is creative, talented, and intelligent? Why did you marry him anyway? If he's that bad, why do you stay married?

You can avoid calling names and flinging out labels if you keep in the forefront of your consciousness the awareness that names and labels oversimplify. You can remember to do this even when you're angry, if you think about it a little bit in advance. It doesn't take a saint to manage this. It only takes a little common sense.

HOW TO LISTEN

Do you think most people are good listeners? I don't. How many people do you know who you feel really listen to you when you talk? Do you feel your husband or wife really listens? Listening is a talent. It requires patience and creativity. The good listener is silent most of the time. But he also must know when to speak. When he speaks he should say something that indicates he has understood what the speaker says. Specialists in communication call this "feedback." The listener should provide feedback to the speaker that communicates the speaker "got through." The speaker then feels encouraged to go on.

Here's an example of an exchange in which the one who is supposed to be listening is not really listening:

Tom: I've been thinking a lot lately about asking the boss if he can use me on a part-time basis instead of full time. I'd really like to head back to school and make something out of myself. This job's just a dead end for me. But I don't know if I should. We might not be able to pay our bills.

Mary: I don't think you should, Tom. How will we pay our bills?

Tom: Forget it.

She didn't even hear his last sentence. She was so busy mentally rejecting the idea that she could not attend to what he was saying. And she missed completely Tom's expression of anxiety and doubt. If she had been listening, she could have merely said, "I see you're concerned about this, Tom." He did not ask for an evaluation. He was expressing a feeling, and his wife failed to understand his feeling. Communication did not take place, and they were both disappointed. Tom was disappointed because Mary did not understand. Mary was disappointed in Tom because she incorrectly believed that he wanted to be irresponsible toward the family.

Try to listen with attention to *everything* your marriage partner says when that partner is expressing a problem or a feeling. Then use the old formula of "counting ten" before you reply. Think before speaking. Say something that indicates that you understood. If you did not get the message, ask for more information.

YOU-MESSAGES COMPARED TO I-MESSAGES

I am indebted to Dr. Thomas Gordon, author of *Parent Effectiveness Training* for the concept of You-messages and I-messages. He applied the concept to parent-child relations. But it is equally applicable to husband-wife relations.

The basic idea is that when another person arouses a feeling in you, it is better to describe your feeling than to fling a character statement at the other person.

Here are some examples of you-messages:

"You never pick up after yourself, Richard. How many times must I ask you to put your dirty socks in the hamper?"

"You're always chattering on the phone with Maxine. Do you realize you were on the phone for twenty minutes?"

The same messages could have been converted to I-messages as follows:

"When I see your socks on the floor it frustrates me!"

"When you talk to Maxine on the phone for more than ten minutes it really bugs me!"

Superficially, the second set of messages may not seem like much of an improvement. But upon closer examination you will see that absolutely nothing has been said about the other person's character. The speaker has merely identified a personal feeling—hardly something that can be disputed. Of course, the other person's disagreeable behavior has been identified. There is nothing wrong with that. But there has been no attack on the other person's ego. The behavior is a fact. And the speaker's feeling is a fact. So the I-message is a vast improvement over the you-message.

IMPROVING OUR WORD ENVIRONMENT

All of the communication guidelines suggested are ways of improving our word environment. If we think about it a moment, we will see that we live in a world of words. We swim in an environment of words the way fish swim in water.

We have all heard, "Sticks and stones may break my bones. But words will never hurt me." But this bit of verse is not true. Human beings have emotional reactions to words.

This is neatly illustrated by polygraph tests. The polygraph is popularly called a lie detector, and it measures at the same time blood vessel expansion, heart rate, respiration rate, and blood pressure. These functions are controlled by the autonomic nervous system, and in most people they are involuntary. When the average man tells a lie there are usually sharp and uncontrollable changes in his nervous system reactions. These show up on the polygraph.

But it isn't only lies that produce sharp emotional reactions. Words with emotional connotations for a particular person will produce the same sharp reactions. Let's assume that we have a subject named Bill hooked up to the polygraph. We slowly read to him the following list of words: butter, chair, horse, Tom, book, dead, pencil, sky, butterfly, Bill, owl, coffee, and telephone. We note that there were sharp changes in the polygraph recordings when the following words were spoken: horse, dead, and Bill. A subsequent interview discloses that Bill was thrown by a horse two years ago. He is still frightened by the thought of riding a horse. The reaction to the word *dead* is understandable. The dread of death is almost universal. Indeed, research using the polygraph indicates that the emotional reaction tends to occur in atheists and religious people alike. One's conscious beliefs about the afterlife appear to have little effect on one's deeper emotional reactions. Bill's reaction to his own name is also understandable. His name is the symbol for his self. It represents his ego. All kinds of positive and negative associations are connected with his name.

So when couples argue or bicker it behooves them to pay great attention to their choice of words. A wife who says, "Drop dead, Bill" in a pique may think little of it. But in her own way she is hexing Bill the same way witch doctors hex voodoo victims. Keep the words at a concrete level. Express your wishes, but not false wishes. Bill's wife probably doesn't want him to die. She wants something else from Bill. She should ask for it. But don't ask the poor guy to die. If she asks him often enough, he just might decide to do it.

Those of us who were overweight as children or adolescents know how much words can hurt. I remember being called "fatso" many times in grammar school. This obviously had a very adverse effect on my self-image, and drove my self-esteem downward. It is very difficult for children to cope with such things. The sensitivity remains in adulthood. I still have a kind of violent emotional reaction to being labeled or tagged in any way. Even complimentary labels irritate me because they oversimplify my personality. If you suffer from a similar kind of irritation, let your spouse know how you feel. Explain the roots of your feeling. Talk about your childhood with your marriage partner. And, of course, don't use labels yourself.

SEXUAL COMMUNICATION AND OVEREATING

There is a very close relationship between sexual communication and overeating. At first this may seem like an odd statement. But think about it a moment. The sexual drive is a basic one. Hunger is also a basic drive. Both involve areas of the body that are called *erogenous zones*. These are areas of the body rich in nerve endings. Freud specified the three basic erogenous zones: the mouth, anus, and the genital area. The mouth is our first erogenous zone. The baby obviously gets a sensual pleasure from sucking, biting, chewing. This also just as obviously carries over into adult life. In adult sexual relations a great deal of sensual pleasure is derived from mouth-related activities that often involve sucking and nibbling. It is not far-fetched at all to say that we unconsciously associate the pleasures of eating with the pleasures of sex.

It is therefore natural to expect that a person who experiences sexual frustration will often turn to food as a substitute gratification. I have seen this so many times in overweight clients that it has become a commonplace observation. I am thinking of Martha G. Martha seldom experienced an orgasm with her husband. She would become very excited during sexual relations, but almost never reached a climax. Here are her words: "Andy really turns me on. I love his body. And I get so excited almost every time he wants to make love. But the only way he can maintain his own sexual excitement is by being very fast about the whole thing. So he usually reaches his climax before I do. Then he won't do anything else. He's done with me and wants to go to sleep. I lay there for maybe an hour or so, and I can't get to sleep. And he's snoring away! It makes me furious. The only thing that relaxes me is to raid the refrigerator. I seem to go crazy. Many times I eat seven and eight slices of bread with peanut butter and jelly. I usually drink a quart of milk. Bloated and half-conscious—I think I've sort of drugged myself—I'm ready to return to bed. I'm beginning to see clearly now that the food orgy is my best substitute for the orgasm I failed to reach."

Martha was helped in two ways. Psychotherapy clarified the connection between sexual frustration and overeating. This insight made her less in the grips of her compulsion to binge when things did not go right sexually. After several sessions her husband agreed to come in for visits, and he learned to be more considerate and concerned with his wife's needs. As noted by Martha in the preceding quotation, he had a problem maintaining his own sexual excitement. His anxieties and self-esteem problems were aired. Martha was surprised to find out he had any. Gradually the couple moved toward a more satisfactory sexual relationship. The improvement in their sexual relationship was an important factor in helping Martha reduce.

Ted R. provides another illustration of the relationship between sexual communication and overeating. Ted frequently wanted sexual relations in the morning before he went to work. More often than not his wife refused. She wanted to continue sleeping and resented being disturbed. For several months he masturbated in the privacy of the bathroom while his wife and the rest of the family slept. But he was disgusted with himself for this activity. He felt it was below his status as a husband. His private conviction was that his wife was being unreasonable. He fell into a different habit pattern. On mornings when he felt particularly rejected, he stopped in at a local coffee shop on the way to work and ordered a double stack of pancakes. He would soak them in syrup and load them with butter. This provided great balm for his wounded ego and also provided a substitute biological gratification. He went to work almost as satisfied and happy as if he had had sexual relations. The only trouble was that he gained ten additional pounds in two months.

Ted's perception of the situation changed by sharing his problem with members of an overweight discussion group. The women in the group helped him realize that his wife's behavior could not be interpreted as a personal rejection. Several of the women in the group indicated that they would react the same way as Ted's wife no matter how much they loved their husbands. As Ted's feelings of personal rejection diminished, he was able to give up his pancake habit in the mornings.

Ted's problems in sexual communication were not isolated from his general communications problems with his wife. Indeed, it is seldom that a sexual problem exists in a vacuum.

It is rare to find a couple that is authentic in their marriage relationship that has a sexual problem. You may have heard the saying, "If the marriage is rocky, there are rocks in the marriage bed." I think there is some truth in this statement. But the implication that a sexual disturbance is the cause of marital problems is a dubious one. This strikes me as a circular problem: What came first, the chicken or the egg? I would venture the opinion that a sexual disturbance in the marriage is in most cases a symptom of a disturbance in the total marriage relationship between two people. Sexual problems are seldom *the cause.* They are usually *the result.*

You can't just hand a couple with sexual problems a list of mechanical techniques. The problem is essentially one of communication at all levels of their relationship. They have to learn how to stop playing games. They have to practice the principles of effective communication. If you have problems in your marriage similar to those discussed in this chapter, don't just put this book aside after you read it. You'll forget the suggestions in it. Keep it out and refresh your memory. Turn to the section on communication guidelines from time to time and try to apply them.

The theme of this chapter has been: Much overeating can be alleviated by an improvement in communication between husband and wife. I have tried to show how games fat people play destroy intimacy between two people. A game-playing marriage is not a real marriage. It is a dull, lifeless affair; an I-it relationship instead of the more satisfactory I-thou relationship. I have suggested ways people can stop playing games, and I have presented a number of communication guidelines. The principles and suggestions offered in this chapter have a sound basis in research conducted by psychologists and students of semantics. Take advantage of this knowledge, and apply it to improve your life.

Chapter 8

How to Help a Loved One Lose Weight

If you are overweight, the odds are you have a loved one who is also overweight. Obesity tends to run in families. As you come to grips with your own weight problem, what can you do for your marriage partner and your children? It is a very frustrating experience to lose weight yourself and see them remain overweight. One client expressed the following sentiment: "It really bugs me now that I've lost twenty pounds to see Jim and the children as fat as ever. It is beginning to embarrass me to be with them now, and I'm ashamed of it. I want to do something to help them. But I really feel helpless. I'm thinner than my daughter now, and I think I'm resisting losing more weight because of her. I hate to show her up. I hurt for her. What can I do?"

Similar sentiments are frequently expressed by clients in psychotherapy and discussion groups. They want to help an overweight spouse or overweight children. It is also very common for a client to have an overweight boyfriend or girlfriend. A client in this category also has problems to deal with. Should he or she marry the overweight person? Should a weight loss be insisted upon before marriage?

HOW WIVES CAN HELP OVERWEIGHT HUSBANDS

Let's say that you have a husband who has gained weight since you married him. He's no longer that slim young man you married. You look at him in distress and wonder if there is any way you can help him. Perhaps you've already tried to help him. And somehow the problem has become worse instead of better. What can you do? Here are some practical suggestions for helping your husband lose weight:

DON'T BE A WATCHDOG

The first principle is: Don't be a watchdog. This was mentioned in Chapter 7, but it bears repeating here. We all want to have personal freedom. When another person decides to become your personal watchdog about anything, you can't help resenting it. If that person is a man's wife, he resents it even more. Men still feel that they should be the lord and master of their households. When their wives reduce their status, men rebel. One way some men rebel and assert their personal freedom is by eating when their wives aren't looking.

PROTECT HIS EGO

The greatest treasure in this world is not gold or jewels. A much more valuable possession is one's self-image. We all want to think well of ourselves. We all need self-respect if we are to go on living. When a person has low feelings of self-worth he is unfit to live with. So, as tempting as it may be at times, don't criticize your husband when he overeats. Run your husband down and you will have a run-down husband. And don't criticize him for the way he looks in a bathing suit. And don't criticize him for the way his belly sticks out. All of these criticisms will be taken to heart if he really loves you—even if he appears to be ignoring you. And he will only have a poorer self-image. He knows he's overweight. He doesn't need you to tell him.

Try very hard to refrain from negative comments about his appearance or his weight. Instead of motivating him to lose weight, they will shoot his self-esteem downward. One of the responses he may have to anxiety arising from lowered self-esteem is eating as a means of soothing his ego.

APPLY THE PRINCIPLE OF POSITIVE REINFORCEMENT

If criticism won't work, what about praise? Will that work? Happily, the answer to that question is a qualified yes. Psychologists call praise a positive reinforcer. It reinforces behavior patterns that are tending in the correct direction. So when your husband *on his own* eats less, eats correctly, or refuses the dessert, take note and let him know in a positive way that you are pleased. If you are pleased, he will be pleased.

A note of caution is in order here. Don't overdo it. Don't praise him every single time you think that a word of praise is in order. If you do this, your husband will get the idea that you are watching his every move—being his watchdog again. Instead, praise on a more or less random basis. Praise only when it is clearly appropriate—and not too often. Praise given too regularly or too frequently becomes meaningless.

DON'T USE SEX AS A MEANS OF CONTROL

One wife told me, "I've got Harry's weight problem licked. I told him no more sex until he loses ten pounds. That should motivate him." Her plan backfired. Harry didn't lose the ten pounds, and after one month without sexual relations the couple had a violent quarrel. Harry lost his temper and hit his wife for the first time.

Actually, the loss of sexual gratification is more likely to motivate a man to overeat than to lose weight. You will recall from Chapter 7 that Freud said the mouth is our first erogenous zone. We are prone to regress in our behavior to this zone when we are sexually frustrated. It is not far-fetched to assume that if a man is denied one kind of bodily pleasure, he will seek another kind of bodily pleasure as a substitute. A man who is sexually ungratified may turn to food as a secondary form of gratification.

Sexual relations in a marriage are an expression of the love and intimacy two people feel for each other. When one person tries to use sex as a means of manipulating another person, the authenticity of the human relationship is destroyed. Of course, I cannot tell you to force yourself to have sexual relations with a greatly overweight husband if such relations have become repugnant to you. However, in my experience this is seldom the case. If it is, then rejection of your spouse is authentic, and not a form of manipulation. However, I am here addressing myself to wives who think they can perhaps motivate their husbands by withholding their bodies. My advice is straightforward. You can't. Don't do it.

COOK SMALLER AMOUNTS

Alice B. is an excellent cook. Not only does she prepare delicious foods, she also prepares large quantities. There are four people in her household—herself, her husband, and two children. Yet she regularly sets out enough food for dinner to feed eight people. Her husband told me, "Who can diet when you've got a cook like Alice? Last night she served fried chicken. She cooked two chickens, and when I saw that large platter I just couldn't resist going back for seconds and thirds."

The quantity of food set before a living creature has a very important effect on appetite. This was demonstrated some years ago with chickens by the Gestalt psychologist David Katz. He found that a certain group of chickens would normally eat fifty grams of grain from a pile containing one hundred grams. However, chickens in the same hunger condition ate as much as one hundred grams of grain when presented with a two hundred gram pile. In other words, the chickens ate twice as much food when presented with twice as much food. They ate about half and left about half. This is a profound experiment. It illustrates that even among animals the hunger drive does not arise from physiological factors alone. The amount of food presented has an effect on hunger.

The phenomenon is by no means limited to chickens. Have you ever overeaten at a buffet, a wedding party, or a holiday just because the food was there? I have—and you probably have too. So take advantage of this principle in helping your husband lose weight. Serve small meals. You may find to your surprise that your husband will be pleased. He's aware of his weight problem too—and he needs all the real help he can get. Just don't make an issue of it. Try to reduce quantities without making a speech about what you're doing.

TRY TO DO LESS SOCIAL EATING

This is difficult to do. But, if possible, try to decline a few invitations that involve eating with other people. The social influence on our appetite is greater than we think it is. Again, the hunger studies of David Katz illustrate this. A first chicken was allowed to peck at a mound of grain until the chicken stopped pecking. Then a second chicken was brought into the experimental room and allowed to peck at the same mound of grain. The first chicken began to imitate the second chicken, and began eating again! This illustrates a second time the principle that hunger is not merely a physiological mechanism. If it is in your control at all, try to find ways to socialize that don't involve eating.

I hope you don't resent the comparison of human beings with chickens. Actually, I have found a way of turning the tables on the experiments with chickens. When confronted with large amounts of food, or when I am in a social situation, I say silently to myself, "I'm not going to act like one of Katz's crazy chickens. I'm not a chicken. I'm a human being." This thought has a way of "short-circuiting" my primitive impulse to overeat. I've suggested this to a number of clients, and many have found it helpful.

BELIEVE IN HIM

Here is a story related to me by an overweight client, Tom L. "The other day Sue and I were in a department store. I tried on a few pairs of slacks, and the only ones that fit were sized at forty-two inches around the waist. Seeing this made me so disgusted with myself that I said to Sue, 'Let's skip it for today. I'm going to get down to at least a size thirty-eight before I buy any more slacks.' What do you think her answer was? She said, 'Oh, Tom, you know you're not going to lose any weight. You've tried before and it's hopeless. Just buy the slacks and forget it.' So we bought the slacks. I couldn't deny that she was right. I've tried to diet so many times and failed. But somehow I feel she should have backed up my good intentions. Only an hour later we stopped in at a coffee' shop and had ice cream sundaes. And I didn't care a bit. I've gained four pounds since that little incident."

It's hard to believe in someone who announces good intentions and then fails to live up to them. But no matter how often your husband has failed to lose weight in the past, when he appears to get interested in weight reduction it pays to support his efforts. This may be the time that something clicks and a real weight loss starts. It is said that hope springs eternal in the human breast. A string of failures in the past does not mean that this time he won't succeed. If hope is killed, then all is lost.

AVOID SPEAKING ABOUT HIS PROBLEM IN FRONT OF OTHERS

It is tempting to make your husband's weight problem a conversation piece. Dieting, calorie counting, and carbohydrate hunting are popular topics at social gatherings. You find yourself drifting from the general to the specific. And soon you are talking about poor Bill's weight problem—the way he's been gaining lately and just can't take it off. Does anyone have any suggestions? Meanwhile, poor Bill is cringing and embarrassed.

You may hope that by embarrassing him and bringing up the problem for public discussion you can motivate him. But this kind of negative approach seldom works. It will only downgrade his self-esteem, and may send him on an eating binge behind your back.

HOW HUSBANDS CAN HELP OVERWEIGHT WIVES

Let's assume you are a husband with an overweight wife. It distresses you to see rolls of fat where there was once a slim little waist. Your wife talks constantly about diets. But nevertheless she seems to get slightly fatter each year. What can you do? Are you just a helpless bystander? The principles involved in helping your wife lose weight are basically the same as those already detailed for the wives of overweight husbands. But let's make some specific applications from your point of view.

DON'T BE TOO DIRECT

You want your wife to lose weight. It is very important to you. The most obvious thing to do is to complain loudly and frequently to her about how fat she is. I know of one husband who nags his wife constantly about her weight. She has told me that it's always on his mind, that he's always putting pressure on her to lose weight. But she's been gaining instead. She breaks the diet when he's not looking. She's the watched dog, and she is striking a blow for personal freedom.

If a husband lets on to his wife that he feels desperate about her weight problem, this may be definitely turned to his disadvantage by some women. Overeating by your wife may be one of her means of expressing aggression toward you. You hate to see her fat. So she gets fat because it hurts you. By now you are aware that this is the familiar passive-aggressive behavior pattern. Many overweight persons have difficulty expressing their aggression in appropriate ways, and they fall into the passive-aggressive pattern as a second-best way of releasing hostility.

SET A GOOD EXAMPLE

In an overweight discussion group one wife said, "Jim is always after me to lose weight. But it's a case of the pot calling the kettle black. Sure I'm overweight. And I should lose some weight. I admit it. But Jim has gained twenty pounds since I married him. He's an attorney, and he thinks by wearing good suits it doesn't show. He's got some kind of idea that because he's middle-aged and successful that he's entitled to be what he calls 'portly.' Well, I don't agree with him. I'm middle-aged too. And I've had three children. I'm not the twenty-two-year-old girl he married any more. But that's what he wants, and I resent it!" This wife's bitterness was natural and appropriate.

How slim are you? Do you rationalize your own weight gain by considering it modest compared to your wife's? Do you say to yourself, "After all, I've got a large frame?" Or, "My dad was a husky guy too." These rationalizations and others may keep you from seeing yourself the way your wife sees you. If you are a normal weight, then you've got some right to talk. But if you have a weight problem yourself—even a slight one—then perhaps you should apply some of the suggestions given in this book to yourself and lose some weight right along with your wife. This good example on your part will help to motivate her. If you look slim and trim, your wife will feel uncomfortable not matching you.

HOW IS YOUR SEX LIFE?

As you know by now, there can be a relationship between sexual dissatisfaction and obesity. As already noted, some wives use sex as a means of control. Men are less likely to do this than women. Nevertheless, there are other ways in which men contribute to sexual difficulties in a marriage. One of the most common complaints you hear from married men is, "My wife is frigid." But when this statement is examined, it can mean a variety of things. It may mean that the wife seldom or never reaches a climax. It may mean that the husband is rejected often when he makes an advance. It may mean the wife experiences no pleasure from sexual relations. An uninformed man tends to blame his wife for frigidity. He often feels that she doesn't love him. Sometimes he thinks there is something wrong with her sexual equipment—perhaps she lacks "female hormones." (The reasons for so-called frigidity are more often psychological than organic. The chances are if your wife was once warm and responsive, lack of response has something to do with the way you relate to each other.)

Many women who are capable of reaching an orgasm have inconsiderate husbands. These husbands think their part is over when they reach a sexual climax. The wife of such a husband complained, "If I reach my climax first, then everything is all right. But if Craig reaches his first, then the lovemaking is over. The first time this happened, he just turned over and went happily to sleep. I couldn't believe it. And he could have brought me to a climax. He knew what to do."

"Did you complain?" I asked.

"No, I was so humiliated I kept my mouth shut. I pretended everything was all right. And I'm still pretending when it happens. Now I'm afraid of hurting his feelings. But I feel so *used* when he does this. I'm afraid it's making me colder and colder toward him, and I don't want that to happen."

Note in this case that it is not only the physiological release of the orgasm that is important to the wife. The husband's lack of concern made her perceive him as selfish and uncaring about her. Men have to realize that in general women have very tender feelings about lovemaking. In spite of all the talk about sexual equality, the double standard still prevails. Psychologically most women are "giving" during sex and most men are "taking." A man who is not aware of this, who does not appear to appreciate the fact that his wife is "giving" during sexual relations, will soon find himself with a cold wife.

The husband who is unconcerned about his wife's orgasm is representative of one kind of problem. Almost paradoxically, there is the other kind of husband—the husband who is overconcerned about his wife's orgasm. This kind of husband makes his wife feel as though she is a sexual failure unless she reaches a climax every time they have sexual relations. The wife becomes overanxious, constantly thinking, "Will I make it this time?" This anxiety interferes with relaxation and enjoyment, and the wife does not reach a climax. The harder she tries to have an orgasm, the more impossible it becomes. As she strives for the goal, it recedes from her grasp. Help your wife to reach a climax if this is what she wants. But don't get "uptight" about it. Both husband and wife should develop a philosophy that the purpose of sexual intercourse is to express love and experience pleasure. In an atmosphere of mutual concern orgasms will be frequent, but not necessarily experienced every time the couple has sexual relations.

Another misconception I have heard expressed by some men is that the wife should reach her climax at the same moment the man reaches his. This idea of reaching a climax together is very romantic. And some men resent their wives for having an orgasm before or after they do. The goal of a mutual climax is only important if someone attaches value to it. I would advise discarding this goal. It is too difficult to always succeed with the required timing. Many couples find it much more convenient and enjoyable to arrange for one partner to reach a climax before the other partner.

All of this may sound very far afield from the subject of helping your wife lose weight. But I assure you it is closely related—much more so than you might think. Remember Martha G. in Chapter 7? She went on a food binge when her husband failed to satisfy her. In other cases the relationship is not so clear. The wife nibbles compulsively during the day with no conscious connection between lack of sexual fulfillment in her marriage and overeating. But the connection is often there. The husband who wants to help his wife lose weight should take a close look at his sexual relationship. He should ask himself, "Is it adequate? What can I do to improve it?"

DON'T TEASE YOUR WIFE ABOUT HER WEIGHT

Sometimes a man may think that if he teases his wife about her weight that this may motivate her to start losing. Let's analyze this. What is teasing? Teasing is a form of concealed hostility. It is usually a veiled insult. Let's say you are guests at a wedding party. Your wife takes seconds at the buffet. She eats two pieces of wedding cake. When she stops eating you smile and with a twinkle in your eye try to tease her in what you imagine is a good-natured manner. "What's the matter, honey? Did you lose your appetite?"

She glares back at you and mutters something beneath her breath.

You laugh. "What's the matter, honey? Can't you take a little teasing? Come on, be a sport!"

What do you think you have accomplished? Have you shown her your sparkling wit? Have you demonstrated your concern for her? Have you motivated her? You can answer all of these questions in the negative. What you have accomplished is a raising of the hostility level between you, and you have only made matters worse.

LET HER TAKE THE INITIATIVE

Actually, there's no way *you* can get your wife to start losing weight. *She* has to take the initiative. Don't ask her to go on a diet; don't plead with her to lose weight. She knows she has a problem, and she probably wants to lose weight on a conscious level more than you want her to. But if you have been reading this book you know that an overweight condition involves motives and habits that are often quite complex. If you try to prod her into losing weight, the odds are that in most cases she will become recalcitrant.

If and when your wife decides that it is time to start losing weight, merely show a friendly interest in what she is doing. Don't give her advice or judge her behavior. Cooperate if she says she doesn't want to go out to dinner. Don't complain that "this stuff is rabbit food." Listen to her if she wants to talk about her diet. But try to refrain from venturing strong opinions. Be at her side with loving concern. But let her do it herself.

HOW PARENTS CAN HELP OVERWEIGHT CHILDREN

"I know that Marie could be the prettiest girl in her high school if she would just lose weight. I've had her on at least ten diets since she was twelve years old. I've taken her to diet doctors. She's taken pills and thyroid extract and pituitary shots. But nothing seems to help. I'm at my wit's end. It's so frustrating! What chance does she have for a good marriage if she stays like this?" The mother speaking was a member of an overweight discussion group. She was only slightly overweight herself.

Another mother in the group spoke of her son. "James is fourteen years old and he's at least forty pounds overweight. He doesn't want to strip for gym. He says it embarrasses him to take showers with the other boys. He says they laugh at him. He's always picked last for any teams. It seems that all he wants to do is sit in his room and read now. I've taken him to four different doctors, but we seem to be getting nowhere."

These parents are expressing the frustration that is common with the parents of overweight children. The quotations illustrate the difficulties inherent in helping an overweight child. Let's assume that your child is overweight. What can you do? What should you do?

EXAMINE YOUR OWN FEELINGS

The first step is to examine your own feelings. You should ask yourself why you want the child to lose weight. Is it because of health reasons? Is it because the child is having a difficult time making a social adjustment? If these are your reasons, then you are motivated by proper considerations.

But some parents have more subtle reasons for wanting their children to lose weight. Oh, the valid reasons are there. But behind the valid reasons there may be unmet neurotic needs on the part of the parent. For example, the mother who was quoted at the beginning of this section said that her daughter Marie could be the prettiest girl in her high school. Doesn't this sound just a trifle suspicious? And later the mother said, "What chance does she have for a good marriage if she stays like this?" Knowing this mother, I am aware that she is projecting her own unfulfilled longings on to her daughter. The mother was a popular high school cheer leader. She married one of the stars on the football team. They were the golden couple when they were dating as seniors. Their other young friends perceived him as someone who would become a famous professional ballplayer. She was perceived as a girl who might become a beauty queen or a movie star. The football star became a plumber, and the potential Miss America became an ordinary housewife. Very understandable feelings of disappointment followed. When Marie was born she soon developed into a very lovely baby. The mother began to have a fantasy that Marie would become all that she might have become. In various ways the child was made to carry the burden of the mother's unfulfilled dreams.

When Marie began to gain a little too much weight at the age of twelve, Marie's mother overreacted. She took her to a weight control specialist, made a big thing out of dieting, and in general made the child overanxious about her eating habits. Marie sensed her mother's overconcern. A mild-mannered cooperative child, she at last had a way of controlling her mother. The whole thing became too much of a "cause," a subject of incessant discussion, and as a consequence Marie got fatter. It became a war between them. Marie began to identify her obesity with having some control over her own life, and in a sense "won" the war.

I have gone into some detail about Marie and her mother because the essential features of the pattern are common. This is not to say that all, or even many mothers want their daughters to become beauty queens. But many parents have a reason for wanting their children to lose weight that goes beyond primary considerations—health and social adjustment. For example, many parents feel ashamed of an overweight child. They feel the child is an affliction. The child's obesity triggers their dormant feelings of inadequacy as parents: *We don't know what we're doing.* This too produces overconcern, and there is an atmosphere of war in the home concerning the child's weight problem.

So ask yourself why you want your child to lose weight. It may be to satisfy needs in yourself such as unfulfilled dreams or ambitions. Or it may be your need not to feel ashamed of your child. Possibly it may be your need to feel adequate as a parent. But any of these seemingly legitimate needs may induce you to overreact and become "uptight" about your child's problem. Emotional scenes with your child will follow, and you will end up doing more damage than good. The first thing you have to learn to do if you really want to help your child is to control your own emotional reactions. The popular phrase that is applicable here is, "cool it."

SHOULD I DO NOTHING?

It may sound like I'm saying, "Do nothing." But, no, that's not quite right. There are quite a few things a parent can do. As already noted in this chapter, a mother can cook smaller amounts of food. Children are like Katz's chickens too. They tend to eat more if they see more. A mother can also serve meals that are low in calories or low in carbohydrates. But she should not call attention to this fact. Obviously, a child has many opportunities to eat when the parents are not looking. If the child feels he is "being put on a diet," he will probably sneak food to make up for what he imagines is a state of deprivation.

Wait until the child complains about being overweight. You may think that you will have to wait a very long time. But this isn't so. If you don't complain about your child's weight, you'll soon find that your child will complain. When your child does complain, offer assistance. Ask, "How can I help? Got any ideas?"

But don't say, "I've been wondering when you were going to ask. This is what I think you should do. . ." You've already turned your child off. As children, they have a great need for autonomy and self-control. And we can only meet that need as parents by understanding their inner needs.

This sounds threatening to some parents. "But I'm the authority!" they protest. That's right. You're the authority. But there is a big difference between being an authority and being *an authoritarian.* An authoritarian tells people what to do and how to do it. This is almost always resented even if it is done in a mild tone of voice and with the best of intentions. An authority, on the other hand, is knowledgeable and a source of information. So you can be an authority. If your child asks, "Say, Mom, how many calories in a teaspoon of peanut butter?" I would provide the answer or show the child where he can look it up. An authoritarian parent won't wait for the question. An authoritarian parent might see the child smearing peanut butter on bread and say, "Do you have any idea how many calories there are in a teaspoon of peanut butter?" The child glares back, insulted. "Sure I know!" Words have been exchanged, but communication has not taken place.

Another important thing you can do is take your child to a physician for assistance with a diet plan, a medical checkup, and so forth. In some cases, you may want to take your child to a psychotherapist for assistance. But here is the key thing: *take the child only if the child wants to go.* Again, wait until your child expresses a desire to lose weight. Medical services and psychotherapy should be made available to the child as a way of cooperating with the child's wishes, not as something imposed on the child.

PRIOR TO ADOLESCENCE

Naturally, helping a very young child is somewhat different than helping an adolescent. Certainly if a toddler has a weight problem, you will want to take the initiative. You can't very well wait until the child expresses a wish to start reducing. In the absence of an organic abnormality, you will want to find ways to restrict the quantities of food you serve and the kind of food you serve. He will probably eat less if he sees less (the Katz principle again). You can switch from whole milk to non-fat milk. Don't keep a lot of cookies, candy, and other high-calorie snacks in the house. But as with older children, don't make too much of an issue out of these things. If you are leaving a restaurant, and the hostess offers your overweight toddler a bit of candy, at that point I would certainly let him have it. He shouldn't be made aware that here is something we can do battle over.

If your child is in the grammar school category, he will almost certainly be distressed by his overweight condition. A boy will be disappointed because he cannot participate successfully in playground games. He'll probably have a nickname such as "Fats." He may smile when called this name, but it will hurt his feelings nonetheless. A girl's self-image problems will be even worse than a boy's. A little fat girl will not feel pretty. Even in grammar school it is very important for girls to feel reasonably attractive. It forms a foundation for the eventual self-image that is stabilized in adulthood. The point is that your grammar school child has good and sufficient reasons for wanting to lose weight. But even at this age you cannot take the reins out of his hands. Tell him he must lose weight, run him around to physicians against his will, put him on diets, don't let him eat desserts with the rest of the family, and you will make the problem worse. You will entrench it.

You must have the patience, even with a child this age, to wait. When the child asks for help, then help. Ideally the whole family should cooperate. If the child is not to have ice cream after dinner, I think it is cruel and unusual punishment for the parents and other children to sit and enjoy ice cream while the child looks on. The child of grammar school age will have sufficient problems with self-control. He needs all the real help he can get. Efforts should be made to enlist the assistance of other children in the family.

THE MOTHER-CHILD RELATIONSHIP

Many a mother starts out by worrying if her child is going to get enough to eat. There is much concern as follows: Will the baby finish his bottle? Will he finish his cereal? Will he finish his dinner? Why doesn't he eat his vegetables? There is apparently little recognition of the fact that a healthy organism—ant, fish, or human being—is highly unlikely to let himself starve to death. We certainly were born with as much sense about eating as an ant or a fish. But the hyperanxiety about eating of many mothers is finally communicated to many children. For these children food becomes overvalued.

Eating becomes too important to the child. The "good child" eats everything on his plate.

If the child starts to become obese, the mother's over-concern about the child's eating behavior continues in a reverse way. Now the child "has a weight problem." (He may be only five pounds overweight.) And so these mothers start in as follows: "Don't you think one helping of potatoes is enough, Johnny?" "No, you can't have an ice cream cone today, Billy. You've had quite enough food for one day." "You are getting to be a very overweight young lady, Sally. Boys won't like you if you become fat, you know." And so it goes. What started out as a minor problem which would have been self-correcting is aggravated by the mother's overconcern.

In the early years, the mother's attitude should be: If he's hungry, he'll eat. Don't encourage a toddler to finish his meal. If he balks, shrug your shoulders and let it go. If he leaves three-fourths of the milk, put the glass in the refrigerator and save it for next time. Toddlers often have little or no appetite at a particular meal. The wisdom of their little bodies is far greater than the wisdom of we adults who insist that they finish what has been set before them. After all, the quantity set before the child was dictated not by the child's inner needs, but by the mother's preconception of the child's appetites and needs. The mother's preconception is a very poor gauge.

If you take this advice, you are likely to have a child with a healthy appetite and no weight problem. The child will like food, but he will not overeat. Food will not acquire exaggerated positive and negative associations. Of course, there is always the possibility of organic and constitutional abnormalities. But in the majority of cases, overweight children are made, not born. They are made by the eating habits they learn from their parents.

IT'S YOUR CHILD'S PROBLEM

As much as you may be distressed by your child's weight problem, you must realize that basically it is your child's problem, not yours. This is very difficult for many parents to accept. "What do you mean it's my child's problem?" they protest. "I'm the one who has to—" To what? To feel embarrassed, inadequate, and guilty? That's right. And that's *your* problem, not the child's. But that's not a weight problem. It is your child who must suffer the direct consequences of being overweight. An obese child has a great emotional burden. Your heart may suffer for your child, but you must not try to carry the child's burden. If you do, you will feel harassed and helpless, and the child will not take responsibility for his own behavior. Back off. Let the child experience the direct consequences of his eating habits. In this manner you will create the all-important conditions for inner motivation.

IF YOUR BOYFRIEND OR GIRLFRIEND HAS A PROBLEM

Some years ago there was a popular song called *The Too Fat Polka:*

> I don't want her.
> You can have her.
> She's too fat for me.
> She's too fat for me.

> I don't want her.
> You can have her.
> Please do that for me.
> She's too fat, she's too fat!
> She's too fat for me!

This song reveals in no uncertain words the kind of rejecting attitude most young men have toward overweight girls.

And, of course, most young ladies have the same rejecting attitude toward overweight young men. And yet one wonders. Why was the singer in the song dating a too-fat girl in the first place? Was she fat when they first met? Did she gain weight later? Although most slim people do not want to date someone who is overweight, it is not uncommon to find a slim person regularly dating a fat person. I have known a number of slim people engaged to marry overweight persons. In several cases I have had these slim people enroll in my psychology of weight control classes, and as a consequence I have gained some insight into how a slim person feels toward an overweight boyfriend or girlfriend.

WHY ARE YOU DATING AN OVERWEIGHT PERSON?

The question a slim person dating an overweight person most frequently asks is, "How can I help my boyfriend (or girlfriend) lose weight?"

I counter with, "Why are you dating an overweight person?" The reason I ask this question is because it is important for the slim person to examine his own feelings before trying to correct someone else's behavior. There are a number of reasons why a person of normal weight might be attracted to someone who is overweight. Perhaps the normal-weight person has a poor self-image for other reasons. People of normal weight often think one or more of the following: My nose is too big, I'm too short, I'm too tall, I'm not well-built, my ankles are too thick, my chin is weak, my cheekbones are too high, my hair is stringy, my breasts are too small, my breasts are too big, I'm knock-kneed, my teeth aren't straight, I'm round-shouldered, my eyes are too close together, my brows are too low, my hips are too wide, and so forth. No matter that an outside observer fails to detect the presence of the problem or thinks of it as very minor. From the inner world of the individual the problem is of some magnitude. As a consequence, the person feels physically inferior and only deserving of someone who is equally inferior. The overweight boyfriend or overweight girlfriend fills the bill.

Under these circumstances, the last thing in the world the normal-weight person wants is for the overweight one to lose weight. Keep in mind that all of this is probably more or less unconscious. On a conscious level, the person of normal weight wants the overweight sweetheart to lose weight. So we come to the concept of *ambivalence,* an important concept in psychology. Ambivalence means feeling two ways about the same person or thing.

This feeling was summarized by Betty G., a girl of normal weight taking a class in the psychology of weight control. "I want Eric to lose weight so badly. He's gained twenty pounds since we've gotten engaged. We bicker about his weight constantly. I've told him he's got to lose the twenty pounds or the wedding is off. But even if he loses the twenty pounds he'll still be fat. When I think of him losing more than twenty pounds I think I kind of panic. I wonder if I'll be able to hold him if he's ever a normal weight. He's so intelligent and basically good-looking that I doubt it."

ARE YOU TRYING TO BE PYGMALION?

Did you see *My Fair Lady?* It was based on the play *Pygmalion* by George Bernard Shaw. Professor Higgins transforms an uncouth girl into a gracious young lady. It is the theme of the ugly duckling changing into a swan. The same theme is the basis of the fairy tale *Cinderella.* The theme has a universal appeal. It is so familiar that it has become a subject of satire: "Take off your glasses, Miss Jones. Now, unpin your hair. By Jove, Miss Jones! You're beautiful!"

To a certain extent, we would all like to play the part of a god. There are women who marry alcoholics with the idea that they will reform them. And so in the same way some persons of normal weight hope to play Pygmalion and transform the ugly duckling into a swan. This is a very unsound basis for a relationship. You will probably fail as Pygmalion, and you will be stuck with something you don't want. Ask yourself if you are really trying to play Pygmalion. If you are, I strongly suggest you consider breaking off the relationship.

PERHAPS YOU ARE PLAYING A GAME

Keep in mind that you may be dating an overweight person because you want to play one of the parts in the games fat people play. It is possible that you want to play the part of *Jack Sprat* and feel superior to your buttercup. Maybe you want to be a watchdog because you have a powerful need to control others. If you're a girl, it's possible that you want to play the part of mommy in *Mommy's Little Boy;* you may have a need for a passive male who can be manipulated with food. If you're a male, you want to be daddy in *Daddy's Little Girl;* maybe you're attracted to an overweight girl because she literally seems a cherub you can possess with sweets. These are all possibilities. If you suspect that any of these motives are operating in yourself, I would take a hard look at your relationship with your plump darling. It may be that your affection grows out of neurotic needs. If so, your affection is bound to deteriorate in the long run. You will end up in the rut of a manipulative game with little real intimacy between the two of you.

HOW TO BE OF REAL HELP

Let's assume that the basis of your relationship is sound. You are drawn toward this overweight person because of mutual interests and values. You "click" together. There is an understanding and a rapport between you that you seldom feel with other people. You have a good feeling toward the object of your affection in spite of the overweight condition. Naturally, you want to see the person become a more normal weight.

The only way to be of real help is to do the things already discussed in detail in this chapter. Don't nag, don't be a watchdog, don't tease, set a good example yourself, avoid speaking about the problem in front of others, try to do less social eating (difficult when you're dating), believe in the other person, and let the overweight person take the initiative. You may wish for more powerful techniques. You want to be able to take direct action. But that is wanting to play God again. You can only help by indirect action.

A young man who took one of my weight control classes had an overweight girlfriend. For two years he had her on all sorts of diets. Every evening he made her account for her day's calories. On the surface, she cooperated. She wanted to please him badly. But she resisted in little ways. She would "forget" to write something down for his perusal, she would go on binges she dared not reveal to him, and so forth. Sometimes she fasted for days at a time. Nothing worked. At the end of two years she was slightly heavier than when they started dating.

Recently I received a note from her. Keep in mind I never saw the girl. Only the young man took the class. Her note said, "I want to thank you for Walter's change of attitude toward my weight problem. Taking your class has made all the difference. Now I feel he's on my side instead of against me. I've lost twenty pounds. Only ten pounds to go and I feel great. Thanks again." Receiving her note was a very gratifying experience for me.

In this chapter I have illustrated how one can help a husband, wife, child, or sweetheart lose weight. The point has been stressed that direct action on your part will usually backfire. We may not like it, but people can often be like mules. The harder you push and pull on a mule, the more unmoving the creature becomes. The mule moves when he wants to move.

You must thus wait until your loved one expresses an interest in weight reduction. You can then offer real assistance when it is asked for. But even when you are asked for assistance avoid too many explicit suggestions, giving advice, and making judgments. Don't give the impression you are taking over. Keep in the forefront of your mind that it really is the other person's problem, not yours. The other person has to learn to deal effectively with the consequences of his behavior.

If you respond in the ways I suggest, you will be perceived as a friend. Communication will flow between you and the loved one. If you persist in behaving in stereotyped and unthinking ways, you will be perceived as an enemy. It will be war, and you both will lose. Apply the principles suggested in this chapter and be perceived as a friend.

Chapter 9

Can Psychotherapy Help?

Throughout this book I have made frequent references to psychotherapy. But what is psychotherapy? What can you expect if you make an appointment with a psychotherapist? Can psychotherapy really help the overweight person?

Psychotherapy is not mumbo jumbo, voodoo, black magic, a dark art, or an occult science. Psychiatrists and psychologists are not members of a priesthood engaged in exchanging esoteric knowledge. Everything that psychotherapists know and use on a technical level is in open stacks in university libraries.

INDIVIDUAL PSYCHOTHERAPY

A great many patients are seen on an individual basis. This one-to-one conversational setting has a time-honored tradition behind it. Freud, Jung, and Adler, the founders of verbal psychotherapy, all saw patients on an individual basis. Usually patients are seen once a week for a "fifty-minute hour." (Some patients in intense psychoanalysis see their therapists once a day. But this is the exception in general psychotherapy, not the rule. Once a week visits are more typical.)

Most of the psychologists and psychiatrists in private practice today are not pure Freudians or straight behaviorists. They are in the main "eclectic"—that is they have attempted to take the best from varying schools of psychology. Thus you can expect a variety of techniques and approaches in your interviews.

FREE ASSOCIATION

One of the classical methods for ferreting out unconscious motives and unconscious conflicts is the method Freud called *free association*. In the free association method the patient is instructed to say anything and everything that comes into his mind. No censorship is to be exercised. And no particular order is to be followed in the presentation.

The instructions may sound easy to execute. But most patients find it difficult to report honestly to a therapist *everything* that comes to mind. What if a female patient is free associating, and what if one of the thoughts that comes to mind is, "Dr. Smith can put his shoes under my bed any time." What will she do? She is probably going to censor the thought and not report it to Dr. Smith. Yet the instructions for free association asked her to report the thought. Other thoughts are brushed aside as unimportant. A patient is free associating and thinks of a day spent alone with father when she was seven years old. He took her fishing, and it was a pleasant childhood memory. The memory seems trivial, and the patient neglects to report it.

Judgments on the part of the patient such as "it's trivial" or "I dare not say that" are all examples of *resistances*. These resistances are thrown up as blocks to self-understanding. The therapist has to help the patient work through the resistances in order to get at their unconscious roots. Thus when a patient hesitates, stumbles, stammers, or chooses words too carefully, the alert therapist realizes that it is very likely a resistance is being encountered. Encouragement and goodwill on the part of both the therapist and the patient are necessary to overcome resistances and in time generate a clear picture of the unconscious motivational structure.

I do not wish to imply that free association is the only method for getting at unconscious motives. As indicated in Chapter 2, straightforward questions can also be a useful device. While not as colorful as free association, they have the advantage of being much more direct and to-the-point. It is, of course, much easier to defend against them and continue kidding yourself. Free association is a way of getting around a rigid ego defense system structure. Nevertheless, in many cases persons can respond to direct questions with insights. The insight may not come the first time the question is asked. But the question will set up a thought process that may lead to a growth experience during the time intervening between visits. This approach was used with success by Alfred Adler.

CLIENT-CENTERED THERAPY

Adler's form of psychotherapy involved face-to-face visits with direct questions and much in the way of human encouragement. The motion-picture stereotype of psychotherapy in which the patient reclines on a couch, and the therapist sits behind the patient, should be reserved only for classical psychoanalysis as first formulated by Freud. Adler's more direct method of an informal face-to-face interview was a precursor of a kind of therapy now called "client-centered therapy." Client-centered therapy is most frequently associated with the name of Carl Rogers, an influential psychologist and theoretician. Client-centered therapy makes the patient's feelings the center of discussion, and the patient tends to take the lead in the conversation. The main role of the therapist is seen as helping the patient clarify his own feelings to himself. Thus the patient may say, "Last night I woke up at two o'clock, and I don't know what got into me. I just had to raid the refrigerator. I gorged myself. And I've been dieting so well for two weeks. But I just went on a binge. This morning when I looked at myself in the mirror I just couldn't stand it. I just wanted to cry. I wanted to break the mirror or break something. Then today at work I just couldn't stand that simpering fool, Jane. She thinks she's a Hollywood dream girl or something—always buttering up our boss, Mr. Wilson. So I let her have it at lunch. I told her what I thought of her—just a pig in my estimation."

The therapist might reply, "It seems to me that you're saying you were angry at yourself, and you took it out on Jane. She was the scapegoat."

The therapist's statement, while both simple and obvious, helps the patient to summarize and clarify her own feelings.

I am not here trying to present a theory of psychotherapy. I am just trying to give you some idea of what you might expect in individual psychotherapy. Free association, direct questions, and a focus on feelings are approaches which you can expect to be utilized by a skilled and versatile psychotherapist.

HYPNOSIS

Overweight people are often very interested in hypnosis as a method of treatment. Unfortunately, they often look upon it as a possible "magic treatment" that will make their weight problem vanish. I have had a number of overweight people ask me, "Couldn't you just hypnotize me and make me hate food?" This question reveals that they are searching for a simple solution to a complex problem.

Suggestions, like seeds, must be planted in a fertile soil. It is not the depth of the trance nor the dark penetrating eyes of the therapist that make suggestions "take root" and grow. It is the preparation of the patient for the suggestion.

Thus if a patient has a number of unconscious motives for wanting to remain fat, then no number of strong hypnotic suggestions are going to override these deeper emotional sources, In a sense, unconscious motives act as hypnotic suggestions themselves. It is absurd to think that suggestions planted by a therapist—suggestions with no "steam" or "drive" behind them—will have any long-range effectiveness.

I do think that hypnosis can be used as an adjunct to conventional psychotherapy. As a person grows in self-understanding, there is no reason he cannot be given a helping hand by the use of hypnotic technique. Suggestions to the effect that certain foods will be unappealing can help the patient get over certain humps.

You might be wondering about the use of hypnosis to get at unconscious motives. Isn't this a way of getting past the ego defense mechanisms? The answer is, yes, it can be used this way. But a number of psychotherapists, including Freud himself, did not find it as effective as other techniques. If, for example, the patient goes into too deep a trance, there is little advantage to discovering an unconscious motive. The whole point to discovering unconscious motives is to make them conscious. If the patient is in a deep trance, then he is not likely to be able to deal too effectively with the recalled material. If you try to get around this by suggesting to the patient he will recall in the post-hypnotic period everything remembered in the trance, there are potential dangers.

Perhaps unconscious material was discovered that the patient is not ready to deal with yet. There is the risk of inundating the patient's ego with a flood of unacceptable material. There is the possibility of precipitating a psychotic reaction or a deep depression. After all, the ego has its reasons for repressing certain motives and conflicts. And the ego will not let the material out until it is ready. If the patient is dealt with in a conscious state, then the ego defense mechanisms can operate in a naturally protective way in psychotherapy.

There is no single royal road to take when dealing with a weight problem. There is no Mandrake the Magician waiting with alchemical hypnotic words to dissolve your fat. Hypnosis can be a useful tool. But it is no cure-all. Beware of charlatans who place ads in the newspapers ballyhooing hypnosis as a semimagical cure for overeating.

FANTASY AND AVERSIVE CONDITIONING

There are suggestive techniques other than hypnosis. One of these is *fantasy*. Of course, it is possible to use fantasy in combination with hypnosis. But it is not essential to hypnotize people in order to induce fantasies. It is quite feasible and efficient to simply ask a patient to relax, close his eyes, and have certain images come to mind. Fantasy can be used in a number of helpful ways in cases of eating problems.

I recall a client, Sally G., twenty-two and single. She worked part-time in a doughnut shop, was a preteaching major at the local state college, and lived alone in a small apartment. She was about eighty pounds overweight the first time I saw her. Her problem was not doughnuts. While working at the doughnut shop she had no trouble with overeating. But on her way home she passed a particular Mexican take-out drive-in, and she had developed a habit of stopping for tacos.

She had already lost over twenty pounds on her own

before coming to see me. And a series of interviews clarified her reasons for overeating. By living alone in an apartment she had already taken a major step toward independence, and in many ways she was and is a remarkably strong person. It was clear that she was well on her way to working out her own problems before she came to see me. Nevertheless, the tacos were a bugaboo. They were a nuisance. I did not think that her yen for tacos indicated a deep unconscious resistance to losing weight. They fell in the category of a bad habit that was self-perpetuating and self-defeating. Under these conditions I could see no reason not to attempt a procedure called *aversive conditioning.*

Aversive conditioning is a form of classical conditioning in which a pleasant stimulus is associated with an unpleasant stimulus. For Sally tacos were the pleasant stimulus. In order to find an unpleasant stimulus, I asked her what she would not put in her mouth under any circumstances. She answered, "snails."

I asked Sally to close her eyes, and a fantasy was vividly described in which Sally was eating tacos filled with snails. It turned out that Sally was very suggestible, and immediately she had a very repugnant image of crunching down on taco shells and snail shells at the same time. We continued the fantasy for about fifteen minutes during the first aversion session. Then we had her experience the same fantasy one week later in a second aversion session. She stopped eating tacos after the first session, and has not eaten a taco since. Here is her reaction to the aversion therapy in her own words:

"I can still see those snails in the tacos. I keep thinking of Dr. Doolittle and the huge snail he had. And the pathetic eyes! I see the snails in the tacos looking like miniatures of Dr. Doolittle's big snail. And they're looking up at me with their wide innocent eyes as I crunch down on them. It's horrible. I could eat tacos if I wanted to, but the whole thing's under my control. And if I want to eat a taco, I just think of the snails and the desire to have a taco goes away."

Sally stopped by to see me six months after her last visit—just to say hello. She had lost forty more pounds and reported that the taco-snail connection was still vivid. She could still use it to stay away from tacos.

I recently saw a client, Mrs. G., who had a problem with hamburgers. When she went out shopping she would have two or three hamburgers, then still have a normal dinner pretending to her husband that she had not had any afternoon snacks. She said she could never quite get her fill of hamburgers. In her case I decided to make *satiation* be the aversive factor. With her eyes closed, Mrs. G. visualized a table loaded with hamburgers. I asked her, "How many do you see in your mind's eye?"

She replied, "Oh, they look delicious. I see about forty delicious hot hamburgers."

"And what time is it? Pretend there's a big clock on the wall. What does it say?"

"Three o'clock."

"All right. And let's pretend you're all alone. No one is going to interrupt you. And you can eat all the hamburgers you want. Okay. Go ahead. Start eating the first hamburger. How does it taste?"

"Oh, delicious. I'm just eating it slowly and enjoying it very much."

"Fine. Now let's say the clock reads 3:10. You're just finishing up the first hamburger. How was it?"

"Good. Very good."

"Do you want another one?"

"Oh, yes. I'd like another one. But I shouldn't. I know I should stop at just one."

"Well, go ahead and have another one. It's all right. Just have it and enjoy it. Go ahead."

"Well, all right. But I know I shouldn't."

"Okay, you're eating it. You're eating it slowly, and you're enjoying it and extracting all of the taste from it. How does it taste?"

"Okay. But not as good as the first one. It's getting cold, and I can kind of taste some of the greasiness. I know I won't want another one after I finish this one."

"All right. Now let's say you're finishing up the second hamburger. The clock now says 3:20. Let's go ahead and start on a third."

"Okay. But I don't want it."

"I know. But go ahead and eat it anyway. I want you to eat it. I want you to get your fill of hamburgers."

"Oh, all right. Okay, I'm eating it. But I'm having a hard time. It's cold and tasteless. I'm just not enjoying it at all. But I'll eat it if you say so."

"Yes, go ahead and eat it. Chew every bite and be very aware of how it tastes and how hard it is to get it down."

We continued in this manner until Mrs. G. had eaten a total of nine hamburgers in fantasy. By her fantasy clock, one and one-half hours had passed. Nevertheless, she reported feeling actually stuffed and completely sick of hamburgers. The aversion to hamburgers created by this one fantasy session lasted more than three weeks. At that time she felt a desire for hamburgers returning, and we had another aversion session designed to make hamburgers unpalatable.

Again, I would like to stress that the aversive conditioning won't work on an unprepared patient. If a patient's resistances are high, if unconscious motives for eating are too strong, these will override any suggestions given. Even if the therapist is successful in creating an aversion to a particular food, the patient will surely be clever enough to find a way around this problem. If the patient's desire to overeat is strong enough, the patient will overeat. Thus aversion conditioning is at best another strategy in psychotherapy. But it is seldom the whole answer to an eating problem.

DESENSITIZATION

It may sound strange to say it, but in a sense many overweight persons have a kind of phobia about being thin. I referred to this before in Chapter 2 when I talked about the fear of the unknown. I said in that chapter that the overweight person is to some extent afraid of the new body image that will result when weight is lost. Also, there may be a fear that certain disastrous things will happen when and if the weight is lost. A wife with a great deal of latent hostility toward her husband may have a dormant fear that she will become involved in an extra-marital affair if she becomes attractive to other men. These fears are usually groundless. Losing weight will in the vast majority of cases improve husband-wife relationships. Nevertheless, these irrational fears tend to crop up in psychotherapy, and they must be dealt with. One of the techniques that can be used to get a patient used to the new body image and also elicit some of the unconscious reasons for not losing weight is called *desensitization*. The technique was pioneered by a psychologist named Joseph Wolpe. Wolpe has made many applications of learning theory to psychotherapy.

The whole idea of desensitization as applied to phobias in general is that people with phobias will seldom give themselves a chance to encounter the feared stimulus. A person with a fear of snakes is certainly not going to pick up a snake. A person with a fear of flying is not going to take a trip in a plane. But the way to get over these fears is to deal directly with the feared stimulus—a snake or an airplane in these illustrations.

So the desensitization technique basically asks the patient to confront his fears in fantasy. A person with a fear of snakes, for example, might be asked to visualize a snake ten or twenty feet away. This will usually be very anxiety-arousing. But the patient will usually adapt or desensitize to this image in a fairly short time. When this image no longer arouses anxiety, the stimulus is brought closer in fantasy. At each stage the patient adapts, relaxes, and becomes free of anxiety. Eventually, in fantasy the patient can pick up a snake, handle it, and feel no fear. Patients who have been desensitized in this manner can usually pick up harmless snakes with no fear. Desensitization seldom is complete in one session. It may take a number of sessions.

The same approach can be adapted to the treatment of overweight persons. The patient is asked to approach a normal weight—the feared situation—in fantasy. At each step of the way the patient relaxes and becomes free of anxiety. Here is a record of such a session:

Therapist: Okay, Carol. I want you to just lean back in the chair. Make yourself comfortable. Close your eyes and relax. Visualize something nice—something soothing and pleasant. What do you see?

Patient: I see an island—pretty palm trees. A blue lagoon. Like one of those old Bing Crosby movies. The sea is calm. The sun is shining. It's very nice.

Therapist: Good. Just relax and enjoy that awhile and go with it. (The therapist remains silent for fifteen seconds.) Okay. Now let's pretend you're home alone. You're home all alone, and you're in the nude standing on your bathroom scale. What do you see?

Patient: The scale says 195.

Therapist: Now let's pretend the scale is in front of a full-length mirror. You look up and you see yourself in the mirror in the nude. Can you describe yourself to me?

Patient: Yes. Well, there I am. A big blob of fat. A cow. I've let myself become a cow. I'm shapeless, and I hate myself for it.

Therapist: Can you describe your body in more detail?

Patient: Yes. Let's start with my arms. They're almost twice as big as they should be. I hate the way they look. And my stomach is huge—enormous—much too big. And my breasts are so fat that they're hanging and weighing me down.

Therapist: Now let's pretend you have a magic button you can press. This button makes you lose ten pounds at a time. If you press the button, you will go down to 185. Do you want to press the button?

Patient: Yes.

Therapist: Okay, go ahead. Press the button and you will lose ten pounds. Now tell me what you experience.

Patient: Okay. I'm pressing the button. (Patient makes a gesture with her hand as if pressing an actual button.) There! I'm ten pounds lighter now. The scale says 185. That's a good feeling!

Therapist: Now describe yourself in the mirror. How do you look?

Patient: Better, but not much. Still a fatso.

Therapist: Any anxiety?

Patient: None! Losing ten pounds only makes me happy.

Therapist: Fine. Let's press the button again and go down to 175.

Patient: Okay. (Presses imaginary button.) All right, I'm at 175 now. I know you're going to ask me to look in the mirror. Hmmmmm. Well, there's some slight improvement. My stomach is a little flatter. That makes me feel happy. And my breasts aren't so fat. They look a little better.

Therapist: Any anxiety?

Patient: Maybe a little. Yes, I'm a little uncomfortable, I think. I don't know why exactly. But mainly I'm happy I've lost twenty pounds. I like the way I look.

Therapist: Do you want to press the button again? Do you want to go down some more?

Patient: Oh, yes! This is fun. I want to see how I look when I'm thinner.

Therapist: Okay. Press the button again. Let's go down to 165.

Patient: (Presses imaginary button.) There! The button was stuck a little that time. I had a hard time getting it to go down. But here I am at 165. Funny, though! I can hardly read the numbers. They're blurred. And I'm having a hard time seeing myself in the mirror. It's not clear. It's like a picture out of focus. And I can't bring it into focus.

Therapist: All right. Don't try to bring it into focus. Just let it alone. It will focus itself.

Patient: Okay. It's coming into focus now. All right. There I am in the mirror at 165. I'm still fat. But I look a lot better than I did at 195.

Therapist: You've lost thirty pounds. How do you feel about this weight loss?

Patient: Good. But discouraged too. I've got such a long way to go. I want to weigh 120 if I'm to really look right. But anyway, getting to 165 is still a big accomplishment. The picture is getting even clearer now. Yes, I do look better! My stomach is much flatter. My breasts are not so enormous.

Therapist: Okay. Go get one of your dresses out of the closet. Put it on. How does it look?

Patient: I'm swimming in it. Hey, this is really great! I can really see how much I've lost now. Thirty pounds is a lot of weight.

Therapist: Okay. Walk out of your bedroom into the living room. Who is there? What happens?

Patient: Okay. In the living room. I find my husband. He's

reading the evening paper—the financial section. He glances up and is sort of startled by my weight loss. He can see how loose the dress is on me.

Therapist: Is he pleased?

Patient: (Answers slowly.) Yes . . . Yes and no. Hmmmm. That's odd. He's pleased and he isn't pleased. In one way I can tell he's happy about it. But in another way I think that he doesn't like the fact that he can't criticize me and tease me for not making a go of my dieting efforts.

Therapist: I see. Anything else happen between you?

Patient: Yes, I think I'm disappointed that he's not making a sexual advance. There! He's going back to the financial news. So I've lost thirty pounds and he's not wining me, dining me, or becoming romantic. It's just another day to him.

Therapist: That's one of the things you've got to face. A weight loss is desirable, but it is not going to work miracles in your style of life. In the long run your relationship with your husband should improve. But you've got to expect some disappointments too. If you expect these disappointments, you won't be thrown by them and tempted to regress into an eating binge. For example, in your fantasy, do you feel like raiding the refrigerator and binging because your husband went back to reading the paper?

Patient: No. I see that he's tired from a long day of work. And he feels comfortable at home. And I can tell that a part of him is happy—really happy—that I've lost weight. No. I don't feel like binging. I want to keep losing weight.

Therapist: Good. Okay. Open your eyes.

The desensitization technique can be a very useful tool in psychotherapy for the overweight person. The technique gets the person used to a new body image. It also spontaneously elicits the patient's conflicts and brings them out into the open where they can be discussed. You will notice that in the technique that patient is not rushed all the way down to a normal weight. It is important to allow the patient to relax and become anxiety-free by stages.

GROUP PSYCHOTHERAPY

Group therapy has been popularized in movies, novels, and nonfiction. *Bob and Ted and Carol and Alice* is a movie that starts with a group therapy experience. *The Lemon Eaters* by Jerry Sohl is an example of a novel that revolves around group therapy experience. And *Joy* by Charles Schutz is a widely read work of nonfiction that describes some of the self-awareness techniques used by group therapy leaders. Assuming the group is led by a skilled and qualified leader, a group therapy experience can be of value to the overweight person. Too often, however, people expect dramatic results in a single session or a single marathon weekend. Instant self-enlightenment is seldom attained. In group therapy as in individual therapy you have to settle down and be prepared to do some hard work yourself.

KINDS OF GROUPS

Groups organized in private practice by psychologists and psychiatrists generally consist of persons with a mixture of problems. In the same group you might find an alcoholic, a young person on drugs, a couple about to be divorced, an individual with a sex problem, and an overweight person. Although these problems may seem vastly different, there is usually a basis for understanding between the members of the group. Here is an example:

Alcoholic: I know why I drink. It all goes back to my fine upstanding father. He always expected too much of me. He wanted me to be a scientist or something. And I couldn't live up to his expectations. So I hate myself. Did you read *My Wicked Wicked Ways* by Errol Flynn? I'm like Errol

Flynn—not as good looking of course. But he was always disappointed in himself because he knew his father disapproved of him.

Drug Addict: Quit blaming your father. Everything you say may be true. But now is now and here is here and he's not the cause of anything now. Man, you got to forget it with all that childhood crap. Just figure it's over. I don't blame my old man for anything. It's *me*.

Overweight Person (to alcoholic): Did your father really expect too much of you? That's interesting. My father was very much the same way.

Therapist (to drug addict): You say you don't blame your father for anything. It's all you. Is this something you're trying to talk yourself into or is it something you feel?

Drug Addict (hesitates and reflects): Good point. I guess I do feel like blaming him. On the other hand, I've been reading some existential philosophers and I'm getting convinced that we've got to stop tying everything to the past. To keep blaming our parents for everything is a cop-out. What about *now?*

Overweight Person (to drug addict): I'm with you. I'm sick and tired of analyzing my childhood. I've had it.

Therapist (to overweight person): A moment ago you expressed interest when Mr. G. (the alcoholic) made a comment about his father. Have you really had it?

Overweight Person (smiling): Another paradox in my nature? Yes, I guess I'm still interested in understanding my relationship to my parents. But I want to go on from that too. Sometimes I feel like a car that's stuck in the mud. I can't go forward. But that's what I have to do. . .

The purpose of the above transcript was merely to illustrate that mixed groups do have something to talk about. And they do learn from each other as they explore their thoughts and feelings in an atmosphere of mutual concern.

Some therapists have organized psychotherapy groups made up entirely of overweight persons. These groups are most often found in public health centers or university clinics. You should be able to find out if there is such a group in your area by contacting your county health office. Generally speaking, however, you will have more trouble finding an all overweight group than a mixed group. If you want to find an all overweight group, you will probably have to turn to some of the self-help groups that have been organized. T.O.P.S. (Take Off Pounds Sensibly), Weight Watchers, and Overeaters Anonymous are examples of such groups that are widely known. You can locate these organizations by checking with your local chamber of commerce. While these groups do not pretend to practice deep psychotherapy, they can often be very helpful to the overweight person in fighting his day-by-day "battle of the bulge." The support and encouragement they give can make the essential difference in some cases. However, if you don't find yourself responding well to self-help groups, then it might very well be to your advantage to seek the services of a psychologist or a psychiatrist.

In this chapter I have tried to show the various ways in which it is possible to employ psychotherapeutic techniques to help the overweight person. I have not tried to "sell" psychotherapy. It helps some overweight people. It does not help others. And, of course, much depends on the particular client-therapist relationship. Sometimes two people just don't "click"—and they get nowhere. I don't think psychotherapy is *the* answer to overweight problems. There is no single answer. A diet prescribed by your physician, reading self-help books such as this one, or joining self-help groups may be all the help you need. But if these approaches to weight control do not succeed, then psychotherapy should be seriously considered.

Chapter 10

Answers to Frequently Asked Questions

People who take weight control classes ask many questions. Some of these questions have a way of cropping up repeatedly in the various classes. They are of interest to almost all overweight persons, and we spend quite a bit of time in the classes dealing with these key questions. The questions and their answers are important because they help clarify a good deal of confused thinking about how to deal with a weight problem.

ARE ALL OVERWEIGHT PEOPLE NEUROTIC?

You might be expecting me to answer this question with a "yes." But we must be careful. To label obese people neurotic is a form of stereotyping that does not do full justice to the psychodynamics of obesity. Although unconscious motives and ego defenses are operative in cases of obesity, they are operative in all people. Actually, a neurotic may be defined as a person suffering from chronic high anxiety. The theory that obesity is caused by an underlying neurosis assumes that overeating is the method a particular kind of neurotic uses to allay anxiety. Although some obese people are neurotic, not all are. When an obese person does suffer from chronic high anxiety, then this is, of course, a compounding factor in his obese condition. But some overweight people are no more anxious, depressed, or frustrated than anybody else. Research by experimental psychologists into the personality structures of obese people shows this clearly. Given the famous Rorschach (inkblot) test, groups of fat people cannot be reliably distinguished from groups of normal-weight people. Actually, the various studies conflict. There is no hard and convincing evidence from the studies that fat people as a group tend to be neurotic. So take heart. Not all fat people are neurotic.

That's the positive side of the coin. This is the negative side: Overweight people tend to use the stereotyped strategy of eating when confronted with depression or anxiety. Although their levels of depression and anxiety may be no higher than normal, they tend to rely on their tried and true formula when depressed or anxious: Eat some food.

It is far too glib to say you're neurotic when you are fat. As a matter of fact, it's a sort of "cop out." It's too easy to excuse yourself for overeating or snacking by saying, "I can't help it. What can I do? I'm neurotic and I need psychoanalysis." What you've got going here is just one more rationalization—an excuse for your behavior. Instead, say to yourself, "Okay. So I'm depressed. What can I do about it other than eating?"

WHAT CAN I DO ABOUT DEPRESSION
OTHER THAN EATING?

We ended the answer to the last question with this new question. Let's not just leave the question hanging. Let's try to answer it. First, remember from Chapter 2 that depression and anxiety often have their roots in unexpressed anger. You want to act in an openly aggressive manner and for various reasons you dare not. And what is making you angry? You probably feel various kinds of frustrations. When you are blocked in your life goals you get angry. So you have to ask yourself what are the sources of your frustration—what blocks you from doing what you want to do in life? Then try to do something realistic about these blocks. If you can't get rid of all sources of frustration—and nobody can—then find harmless outlets for your aggression.

Here are some examples of possibilities other than eating:

1. Write a murder mystery. This doesn't require writing talent. You're writing it for self-expression, not for sales purposes.

2. Paint a picture of a monster. Make it as horrible as you can make it.

3. Hit a punching bag. If you dare, think of the person you really want to hit while you are hitting the bag.

4. Play the part of a villain in a local theatrical production.

5. Take a towel and wring it hard when you would prefer to wring somebody's neck.

6. Make an ugly face in the mirror when you are alone. Say out loud what you are burning to say to your boss, sweetheart, or spouse.

7. Get some play dough and work it into any shape that pleases you. Manipulate it and control it as you feel manipulated and controlled.

8. Play some primitive music when you are alone. Make up your own savage dance to the music.

Perhaps you get the idea. Give vent to some of your aggressions in a nondestructive way. You may think that some of the above suggestions are childish. I assure you they are not as childish as stuffing yourself with food. We all have a child in us that needs a certain amount of expression. You can let that child eat when he gets mad. Or you can let him have a variety of nonfattening expressions. What is better?

ARE APPETITE DEPRESSANTS HELPFUL?

Appetite depressants are frequently prescribed by some physicians. Obviously, there is a widely held view that they are helpful. My own view is that they are only helpful in the short run, not in the long run. My reason for saying this is that appetite depressants act on a physiological level. A person loses his appetite. His craving for food is *suppressed*, not changed. The basic attitudes and habits are still there waiting to come back when the person stops taking the pill. One client, Joan T., weighed 220 pounds. She took various kinds of drugs to control her appetite for one year, and dropped down to 120 pounds. After she stopped the pills, she gained the hundred pounds back in six months. These events transpired before I saw her. When she came in for counseling she was a very discouraged young girl. The experience of losing the weight and then gaining it all back had made her feel that her condition was really hopeless.

She later said this to an overweight discussion group: "I see now that taking pills was a kind of reliance on magic. I wanted the pills to do my work for me. All the time I was taking the pills I kept thinking how nice it would be when I could stop taking them and go back to normal eating. I didn't have much of an appetite because my nervous system was drugged. But I kept thinking about food nonetheless. The devil in me had been locked up. But all the time he was screaming to be free! When I stopped taking the pills I felt as if I had been let out of jail. I ate like there was no tomorrow, and here I am fat again."

Actually, most of the people in my overweight classes have tried appetite depressants one or several times. Very few of these people have found them to provide any kind of real solution to their basic weight problem.

SHOULD I LOSE SLOWLY OR RAPIDLY?

The crash diet has a great deal of appeal. Advertisements in magazines scream about miracle plans that make the pounds vanish in a few days. When an overweight person decides to lose weight there is often a great impatience about the whole business. The weight must come off *now!* There must be no dilly-dallying. It makes no difference that it took several years to acquire the weight. The decision to lose weight is usually accompanied by an impatient enthusiasm. After a few days of deprivation, the flame of enthusiasm begins to sputter. In a few more days it is dead, and the former zealot is back to compulsive eating. "I can't lose weight," he mourns. "It's hopeless. I'm doomed to be fat."

Even if the crash diet works, it is very much the same situation as the appetite depressants. Tom C. lost forty pounds by crash dieting. His eating would have done an ascetic proud. Cottage cheese was the mainstay morning, noon, and night. And he hated cottage cheese. When he lost the forty pounds his attitude was, "Great! Now I can go back to normal eating." In a short time he was heavier than when he had started his crash diet.

One of the troubles with the crash diet is that it puts you into a state of suspended psychological animation. You don't reeducate your eating habits. You're in limbo. When you get out of limbo you're in the same psychological spot you were in when you started dieting. It's no wonder the weight comes back on.

When you reduce too rapidly you don't make the proper psychological investment in your weight loss. It takes place by a "trick." There is very little of "you" involved. You have not had to think things through in terms of your motives, your attitudes toward food and your basic eating habits. As a consequence, it is hard to identify with the new body you have acquired. The less you have of yourself invested in losing weight, the more likely you are to gain it back.

Another flaw in losing weight too rapidly is that it is not good for your health. The odds are that if your diet is too restricted in total calories, you will not get adequate amounts of protein even if you are eating a high-protein diet. This will do damage to muscle tissue and your internal organs. You have seen the drawn, dissipated look that some dieters have. This is frequently due to an imbalanced intake of foods.

So I counsel patience. Be satisfied with a weight loss from one to three pounds a week, depending on your height, present weight, and sex. As long as you can see reasonably steady progress, be satisfied.

WHAT ABOUT "DIET FARMS"?

A so-called "diet farm" is a place people go to remove themselves from the everyday temptations of food. The farms usually have a resortlike atmosphere with comfortable rooms, a swimming pool, various kinds of recreation, exercise classes, and so forth. Usually meals totaling no more than 800 or 1,000 calories are served. No other food is available. The firms tend to cater to women married to prosperous men. Although men are also welcome guests, the women are the backbone of the farms. The stay is usually quite expensive. It is not unusual to pay $200 a week or more.

If you can afford the stay, and if you want to get away from your family for a few weeks, I have nothing to say against the farms on any general basis. But, on the other hand, I'm not particularly enthusiastic about them as a basic solution to a weight problem. Perhaps for a woman who has slowly gained five or ten unwanted pounds the stay at the farm will be helpful. She does not have a serious problem, and her basic eating habits are good. But if you are a person who has been battling the bulge off and on for some time, I don't see how a stay at a diet farm is really going to change anything. Certainly no real deconditioning takes place. You will recall from Chapter 4 that deconditioning takes place *only in the presence* of the conditioned stimuli. In the final analysis, you must extinguish your bad eating habits in familiar surroundings. If you go to a diet farm and lose a few pounds, the odds are at least fifty-fifty that you will gain the weight back when you return home.

Here is how Mildred V. described her diet farm experience to a weight control class. "It was great in some ways. I felt so pampered and so special. The fact that we were getting only 800 calories a day seemed unimportant. The food was prepared and presented in unique ways. We had three meals and three snacks a day. So we were eating all the time. We had exercise classes, and even classes in yoga—which I found fascinating. And I made several new friends. We had some lectures on nutrition, and they were good. Being free of the responsibility of the children for two weeks was an unusual and I must admit somewhat delightful experience. But I missed them and called them every few days. My mother stayed at my house. The whole thing was a birthday present from my husband who will do almost anything to help me lose weight. It cost him $500 for the two weeks. But I guess he felt it was worth it when he saw me arrive home glowing with a positive mental attitude and ten pounds lighter. He treated me to a good dinner out the very next night as my reward, and I started to gain some of the weight back right then. This was all six months ago, and I weigh only slightly less than when I left for the farm. All in all I can't say it made much difference either way. I wouldn't say don't go. It depends on the person. One of the girlfriends I made there took off eleven pounds and she has lost eight more pounds since she's come home. The lectures on nutrition and the yoga classes inspired her. She's taken up yoga as a regular thing now, and I must admit that she has a lovely body."

DO OVERWEIGHT PEOPLE SUFFER FROM A LACK OF CHARACTER?

No one suffers from a lack of character. Everyone has a character. Character may be defined as your distinctive qualities or traits. However, as most people use it, the phrase, "lack of character," probably refers to the lack of a particular trait called *moral fiber*. Moral fiber tends to be associated with the ability to resist all kinds of temptations. If you have moral fiber, then you also have willpower, self-control, and so forth. If you don't have moral fiber, then you will presumably become an alcoholic, a drug addict, a thief, a prostitute, or obese.

This way of looking at human nature seems like a dead end to me. It describes, but does not analyze. If an overweight person complains to me, "I guess I just lack character," I want to know *why* he lacks character. Does he lack character in all respects? Can he resist no temptations? The odds are very high that the client has all kinds of self-control in many life situations.

Concepts such as character and moral fiber stem from a prescientific psychology when philosophers believed that people were born with inborn traits. You carried your traits around in the basket of your personality the way farmers carried eggs around in baskets. The eggs were just there. There was little you could do about them. Scientific psychology presents convincing evidence that most traits are learned. Consequently, there is hope. They can be unlearned. You are alive and changing constantly. Don't fall into the pit of describing your personality in negative terms such as, "I have no character," or, "I have no willpower." Analyze instead. *Why* do you behave as you do? What are your underlying motives? Are you playing games with someone? How can you deal with your ego defense mechanisms? How can you change your habits? These are the things I have encouraged you to do in this book.

ARE OVERWEIGHT PEOPLE A NEW MINORITY GROUP?

Although many people want to lose some weight, there are relatively few people who are very fat. I won't try to define "very fat" with any precision. But you certainly know what I mean. A very fat child is obviously on the outside of things. A very fat adult is clearly visible to all of us. These people probably constitute no more than ten to fifteen per cent of our population. And they certainly do constitute a minority group in every sense of the word. They are often rejected and treated like members of racial and ethnic minorities.

The *Too Fat Polka* quoted earlier was an example of the kind of rejecting attitudes expressed toward very fat people.

Fat children are laughed at and insulted in school. Fat people are indispensable in certain kinds of comedy. They are usually the victim of a slim person's manipulations. I remember as a child hurting with laughter as the slim Bud Abbott made a fool out of the fat Lou Costello.

We often laugh at what we unconsciously·hate. The target of laughter, the butt of a joke, is often a scapegoat for our aggressions. At a repressed level of his personality, a person of normal weight hates a fat person. Why? Because the overweight person symbolizes what the normal person might become. There is an animal fear triggered in the deepest recesses of the personality: *My God, it might happen to me too!* All of this is quite irrational, of course. But that doesn't mean it's not there. The same kinds of feelings exist toward dwarfs, cripples, people with a cleft palate, and persons with other physical abnormalities.

As a consequence of all this, it is difficult for a very fat person to get a new good job, to get promoted, to marry someone desirable, to be accepted in many social circles, and to be taken seriously in general. If you are very fat, you are already aware this is so. You do not need me to tell you. But perhaps you did not know why fat people are rejected. It is worthwhile having some insight into the motives of other people. Rejections lose some of their sting if you can comprehend that the person's behavior is itself rooted in unconscious motives. The attack upon you is not personal. It is representative of a universal trend in human nature: a fear and a hostility toward the abnormal.

I am emphasizing this because one of the overweight person's greatest problems is self-esteem. When others laugh at you or reject you, it hurts and your self-esteem suffers. One way of soothing your wounded ego is to eat something. However, if you can adopt a more understanding attitude yourself, if you can comprehend the other person's behavior in terms of a psychological principle, you will not feel as hurt. You will then have less need for the balm of food.

WHAT IS THE BEST WAY TO SATISFY YOUR HUNGER FOR A SNACK?

One of the greatest problems you have to face is the problem of between-meal snacking. Many overweight people who try to diet decide to completely eliminate between-meal snacking. For a few days they are able to override their craving for something to eat between meals. But it is seldom long before they are back to snacking again. There is a feeling, "I've blown it." And the entire effort to lose weight is undermined.

If you hunger for a snack, I think you should go with your impulse and have it. But you should not eat what you have been eating in the past. Cookies, cake, candy, tacos, ice cream cones, and so forth do not make good snacks. They do not make good snacks for two reasons: (1) they are too fattening, and (2) being high in starch or sugar they stimulate your pancreas to secrete insulin to burn up the sugar. This has a tendency to produce a state known as *hypoglycemia* or low blood sugar. That's right, a high-sugar snack will actually make you hungrier in the long run. In an hour or so you will be craving food again.

You can see from the above paragraph that not all of the abnormal craving for food of the overweight person is psychological. Because the American diet is so high in carbohydrates and refined sugar there are probably many overweight people suffering from mild to severe hypoglycemic conditions without knowing it. Under these conditions your craving for a snack actually has a basis in physiological hunger.

You probably know if your hunger for a snack is mouth hunger or real hunger. When it is mouth hunger you know that you are not really hungry, you just want to put something in your mouth to satisfy your oral craving. When it is real hunger you may feel a little weak or empty in your stomach.

If it is mouth hunger, then return to the principle of stimulus substitution discussed in detail in Chapter 6 on creative weight control. Do your best to channel your oral craving in the direction of very low-calorie or calorie-free foods.

If it is real hunger, it is probably best to eat a high protein snack: cheese, milk, an egg, or some meat. This will have a tendency to satisfy you for a fairly long time.

CAN YOU CONTROL APPETITE WITH
CELLULOSE WAFERS?

Cellulose wafers work on the principle of stimulus substitution. They have no food value, and they are something you can stuff into your mouth when you are hungry. Liquid taken with the wafer makes the cellulose expand, and this in turn distends the stomach. They can be helpful in some cases when there is abnormal mouth hunger. They will give some satisfaction to your oral craving. But they won't do anything for real hunger because they won't do anything to your blood sugar. Again, if you feel you are really hungry, try a high-protein snack.

WHAT ABOUT JOGGING FOR THE
OVERWEIGHT PERSON?

I will respond to the question as a psychologist. I do not claim to be an expert on a medical basis. You might read

Aerobics by Kenneth Cooper for physiological information. Aside from the medical aspects of jogging, I have met very few overweight people who will keep up a jogging program. They often feel embarrassed—and they just plain hate to run anyway. Seeing as most overweight people like to ride I have suggested bicycling as an alternative. Of course, the usual precautions must be given: Build up slowly and don't over-exercise. Mild exercise at first is the standard recommendation. Another form of excellent exercise that many overweight people take kindly to is swimming. People with excess fat are unusually bouyant and are often excellent swimmers. If you fall into this category, I encourage you to swim more. Recent studies by physiologists such as Jean Mayer of Harvard University have suggested that the importance of exercise in weight control has been under-emphasized. Activity is helpful for burning off fat and for keeping it off. (Also, it appears that moderate exercise has a beneficial effect on appetite. Instead of making you more hungry it actually makes you less hungry!)

The problem, however, from a psychological point of view is a lack of desire to exercise that is so common to overweight persons. If you will not exercise more, then you have no choice but to eat less if you want to lose weight. Once again the problem becomes psychological in nature, and the topics discussed in previous chapters of this book become relevant.

From the psychological point of view the essential thing in a successful exercise program is simply this: The exercise should be fun. In view of the fact that very few people think of jogging as fun, it is doubtful that many people will keep it up for any length of time. In contrast, a greater number of people associate riding a bicycle or swimming with fun. Consequently, they are much more likely to keep up these activities over a period of years. Naturally, I am not excluding golfing, bowling, sailing, or other sporting activities. But

I think physiologists who have specialized in studying the benefits of vigorous activities such as bicycling or swimming favor them over golfing, bowling, or sailing.

CAN SELF-HYPNOSIS AND AUTOCONDITIONING HELP ME?

Self-hypnosis involves putting yourself into a trance. The purpose of this is to narrow your attention and make you more susceptible to suggestions. I have indicated in previous chapters of this book that I am somewhat dubious about the use of hypnotic techniques without professional supervision. I wouldn't go overboard on esoteric techniques. Once again, we have the search for magic. The technique, in this case self-hypnosis, is supposed to solve the weight problem. When an overweight person says to me, "Can't you hypnotize me or teach me to hypnotize myself so I can lose weight?" what they are really saying is, "Wave a magic wand and make my fat go away." I dealt with this point at greater length in the chapter on psychotherapy.

Actually, what you really want from self-hypnosis is not the trance but the beneficial suggestions. You need not go through an elaborate trance induction ritual to place yourself in a receptive mood for suggestions. Sit in a comfortable chair, close your eyes, insure freedom from distractions, and this is about all you need to do. You can now recite to yourself previously memorized thoughts of a positive nature. We might call this procedure *autoconditioning* to contrast it with self-hypnosis. Here are some messages you can memorize and recite to yourself in a relaxed state:

1. *A message of hope.* This is a message of hope. I want to start believing that I really can lose weight, and that I really can keep it off. Even though I have tried to lose weight

several times in the past, and failed, this does not doom me to permanent failure. There is a saying that goes, "Try and try again." Very few things are accomplished on the first try. The past does not completely control the present. Many people have lost weight, and I can succeed too. I must believe in myself.

2. *A message about heredity.* I didn't inherit fatness. I may have inherited a tendency toward being overweight. But a tendency is not overweight itself. Many people with a tendency toward being overweight have slim bodies. I am not locked into a hereditary pattern I can't escape. If I change my habits in a healthful direction, I can lose weight and keep it off.

3. *A message about husbands.* I must not blame my husband for my weight problem. Even if he does frustrate me, this doesn't mean I have to overeat. There are better ways to deal with frustration and aggression. It's too easy to blame someone else for my problem. I must remember that "I am the master of my fate. I am the captain of my soul."

4. *A message about wives.* I blame my wife for being overweight because she cooks rich foods and sets an ample dinner table. This is not realistic. She does not actually open my mouth and stuff the food down my throat. I can eat in moderation even if she fixes an ample meal. She won't curl up and die if I refuse her food.

5. *A message about tomorrow.* I say that I will start dieting tomorrow or in a few weeks when conditions are better. I say that I am in a time of stress now, and this is no time to start trying to lose weight. This is not realistic. All times are times of stress. Just being alive is stressful. Now, today, is the time to start bringing my weight problem under control.

The messages suggested are only examples of the kind of suggestions you can give yourself. I would urge you to make up messages of your own which might be even more appropriate to your particular life situation. Write out a message—not too long—perhaps fifty or one hundred words. It should be something you can really believe in. Just thinking about the message and what to write will in itself be helpful. Your involvement in the creation of the message itself will be of value. Commit the message to memory. Then consciously and deliberately recite it to yourself in a comfortable chair with your eyes closed.

Remember that repetition is one of the important keys to learning. Think of yourself as learning a new idea, a new viewpoint. You cannot expect to learn it and make it a part of yourself in one trial. You might find it necessary to repeat messages to yourself for days and even weeks. Even if a beneficial effect begins to take place relatively soon, repetition is still necessary in order to reinforce and maintain the effectiveness of the message. After all, you probably have a lot of past negative thinking to overcome. So stick with it, and give the suggestions a chance to take effect.

There are variants on the autoconditioning technique described that you might consider trying. You can tape the messages on a tape recorder. Play them back to yourself as you relax with your eyes closed. Another possibility is to copy the messages many times, thinking of their meanings as you copy. All of these approaches will help the messages make an impression on you.

DO LIQUID DIETS MAKE PSYCHOLOGICAL SENSE?

Many overweight people find it easier to stick to a liquid diet than to restrict their intake of solid foods. Psychologically, solid foods are temporarily "off limits" and they present no great temptation during the weight loss period. This suggests that many overweight people think like alcoholics. They are "foodaholics." It's all or nothing at all.

Aside from the fact that liquid diets may not be nutritionally sound, they really don't make psychological sense in the long run either. You probably realize by now that very little deconditioning or relearning could take place under the conditions of a liquid diet. The old eating habits remain unchanged, and they usually reappear full-blown and stronger than ever at the first opportunity. I have seen a number of overweight people lose weight rapidly for a few weeks on a liquid diet. They usually gain the weight back just as rapidly when they go off the diet.

DOES FASTING MAKE PSYCHOLOGICAL SENSE?

The psychology of fasting is very much like the psychology of the liquid diet. It is often easier for an overweight person to go on a fast than to eat in moderation. Complete abstinence from food until you are a normal weight makes neither psychological nor medical sense. It has been tried on an experimental basis in some research hospitals with patients described as "superobese." They lose weight during the fast. But they almost always gain it back when they are released from the hospital. It can only be justified as a heroic measure in cases of extreme obesity.

A variant on the total fast that has been tried is fasting on alternate days. Some research reports indicate good results with this method. It seems that "foodaholics" can abstain entirely from food every other day more readily than they can eat in moderation every day. This is very similar to the on-off approach discussed in Chapter 6 on creative weight control. I hesitate to recommend alternate days of fasting because it seems unsound on a nutritional basis. Psychologically it makes some sense, but I would suggest you obtain a physician's approval before trying it.

WHAT IS AN ORAL PERSONALITY?

An oral personality is an individual who obtains an inordinate degree of satisfaction from activities associated with the mouth. An oral personality may eat too much, may also be a heavy drinker, a heavy smoker, or he may talk too much. Any one or all of these traits may be exhibited by a person with an oral personality. You will recall that Freud said the mouth is the first erogenous zone. Psychoanalysts hold that an oral fixation develops if there is a psychological blow that creates a strong emotion during the oral period. The oral period would be the period of infancy and/or early toddlerhood. A commonplace example would be being weaned too early and against your will. Let's say that your mother decided to take the breast or the bottle away from you on some arbitrary basis. At ten months she threw your bottles away and announced, "You're a big boy now. You don't need your bottle any more." Perhaps you screamed, cried, threw a tantrum. But all to no avail. Your beloved bottle never returned. But unconsciously you never forgot. And so you developed an oral fixation. If all of those things really happened, it is not far-fetched to suppose that you might yearn to return to oral gratifications of various kinds during times of stress. This is termed *regression*, and it means returning to an infantile level of functioning. This is why compulsive eating is sometimes thought of as regressive behavior, the expression of an infantile wish to return to the breast or the bottle.

Assuming that this wish does indeed exist in some overweight people, it is clear to see why the principle of stimulus substitution makes sense. It is almost impossible to completely deny an intense oral craving. But it is possible to learn to exhaust its energy on something nonfattening.

WHAT IS THE "VACATION SYNDROME?"

What I am about to write belongs properly to the chapter on the ego defense mechanisms because it is really a special case of rationalization. Nevertheless, it is such an important phenomenon in its own right that perhaps it merits special attention. I am referring to what I call "the vacation syndrome." Have you ever noticed how often people come back heavier from a vacation? One woman I know can come back from a two-week vacation ten pounds heavier. She does it almost every time. Here is her own version of her experience: "I think I go kind of crazy where food is concerned when Fred and I go on a vacation. We like to stay at luxury motels with modern coffee shops. At home I usually have a very light breakfast. But when I'm on vacation I have a complete breakfast every morning. It's as if I've been set free from a prison or something. I'm kind of like a drunk that's fallen off the wagon. I love pancakes—and I know how fattening they are—but I order them at least half of the mornings when I'm on vacation. Then dinner is another big hazard. Fred and I like to go out to some of the better dinner houses on our vacations. So almost every night it's prime rib or steak and a baked potato loaded with sour cream. I eat it all plus the bread that goes with it. And the funny part of it is that I only half-enjoy myself. I'm always vaguely dissatisfied because I know there's a part of me that hates what I'm doing. But all the while I'm thinking, 'After all, I'm on vacation. This is our vacation and we waited all year for it.' When I get home and see I've gained five or ten pounds I'm shocked. I can't believe it. I didn't think somehow that I would actually gain the weight."

This last comment illustrates the great danger of the vacation syndrome: In some distorted way the vacation creates the illusion that all normal processes are suspended. In the same way that the normal day-to-day activities of cleaning house, seeing the children off to school, paying bills, and so forth have in fact been momentarily suspended, the compulsive eater thinks that the laws of nature—in particular the law of metabolism—have been suspended. Unfortunately, they have not. Thus we have the unexpected shock when the vacationer returns home and finds the large weight gain.

The only antidote I know to the vacation syndrome is to produce a counter-thought when you start to think, "I'm on a vacation after all." Instead deliberately think, "I'm on vacation. That's true. But the laws of nature have not been suspended. They're still operating. And I'll gain weight if I overeat." I have gone so far as to suggest to one client that she write down the above sentence on a piece of paper. She was to carry the paper in her purse throughout the vacation. When tempted to slip, it was suggested that she take the paper out and read it. The client reported after the vacation that just knowing the paper was there was enough to make her think of the key sentences written on it. Thinking of these key sentences inhibited the rationalizing thoughts that arose when she was on the vacation.

WHAT IS "NORMAL" EATING?

It is common to hear an overweight person say, "I eat like a bird. But everything turns to fat." Others say, "If I eat normally, I gain weight." It seems to me that there is some confused thinking going on here. Assuming your problem is not an endocrine disturbance, you are either eating too much or eating incorrectly. The only possible definition of normal eating for you that can make sense is eating in such a way that you do not gain weight. Too many overweight people trying to lose weight think, "Just three more weeks of this suffering. And then I can eat normally again." When so-called normal eating resumes, weight is gained. When you succeed in losing weight, you are not released from correct eating habits. Normal eating does not mean you can eat anything and everything you please. Normal eating means making intelligent choices and eating sanely.

CAN AN EX-FAT PERSON EVER RELAX COMPLETELY?

For the majority of ex-overweight people this question has to be answered, "No." Even if your basic attitude toward food improves to the point of being close to a normal one, there is still a residual tendency toward obesity in the majority of cases. In our society only a small percentage of people are an ideal weight (which is, by the way, somewhat less than the average weight published on normal weight charts). Let's face the simple fact that in the United States in the twentieth century most of us get too much to eat. Food is too available. This fact combined with the lack of vigorous exercise demanded to burn up excess intakes of food tends to make more than one-half of Americans weigh more than their ideal weights. So if you want to be thin and stay thin for both physical appearance and good health, it is doubtful that you can ever relax your vigilance.

WHEN IS THE BEST TIME TO MAKE GOOD RESOLUTIONS?

Have you ever noticed how just after finishing a large meal you will be angry with yourself for overeating? Then you make a resolution: "Okay. From now on I'm going to watch it. Next time I won't overeat." But next time you overeat again. Making good resolutions right after finishing a large meal is like locking the barn door after the horse has gotten away. If you're going to make resolutions, make them just *before* you start the meal. Say to yourself, "Okay. This time I won't overeat. I'll skip the second helping and have only one slice of bread." Say this to yourself very firmly and it just might work.

WHAT KIND OF A DIET IS THE BEST?

I do not pretend to be an expert on nutrition. I try to advise only in the psychological realm. It is my belief that most overweight people have tried a number of diets. Usually they have found one or several ways of eating that successfully take off pounds. The problem is usually sticking to a correct way of eating. Excellent menu plans can be obtained through the Weight Watcher's organization, Take Off Pounds Sensibly, government and university departments of nutrition, and your physician.

I am invariably asked what I eat. I avoid sugars and starches. I seldom accept desserts of any kind. I eat very moderately such foods as macaroni, bread, pancakes, muffins, pizza, potatoes, rice, and other starchy foods. I try to satisfy my appetite mainly with meat, fish, vegetables, milk, cheese, juices, salads, and fresh fruits. And that's about it. Basically it is a high-protein, low-carbohydrate diet. I don't count calories even when I am trying to take off a few pounds. I just cut down on sugars and starches. If I get careless on desserts and starches, I usually start to gain again. I certainly don't recommend this way of eating for everyone. It works for me, but it may not work for you. If you have any quantity of weight at all to lose, it is best to do it under a physician's supervision.

This chapter was based on questions frequently asked by overweight clients. I have offered observations and advice based on my experience with these clients. Of course, general advice cannot possibly apply with equal validity to every reader. But I believe that if you select in accordance with your own idiosyncracies, you may find something of value in the preceding pages. The observations and advice are intended to stimulate your own thought processes. The psychology of weight control is a complex topic, and only a fool would assert that he has *the* advice for all overweight people.

Chapter 11

Human Freedom and Weight Control

A client in a weight control discussion group is speaking. Her name is Connie G. She could be a pretty woman, but she is forty pounds overweight. She always keeps her coat on to conceal her body. At this moment she leans forward and speaks intently to the group. "In the end I think we're all creatures of habit. I can't seem to break out of the same dull routines. I find myself nibbling forbidden foods between meals when I've told myself a thousand times I'll never do it again. Sometimes I feel like a fly caught in a web. I keep struggling to break free but I can't. I see now that the web is my unconscious motives and my habits. I guess I'm just stuck with myself the way I am."

Before Connie loses weight it will be necessary to convince her that she is merely uttering one more rationalization.

Another client in the class answers her, "I used to feel the way you do. But I decided I was excusing myself too easily." Connie barely hears the comment.

The aim of this chapter is to convince you that *you are free*. There is nothing in the principles of motivation and habit that make you a helpless victim. As a human being, you are free to respond to your urges and compulsions in a variety of ways. It is the lack of belief in your own power of assertion that is the ultimate source of your difficulties—not your motives and habits.

The great philosopher-psychologist William James fell into a deep depression as a young man. The disease was caused in a sense by knowing too much philosophy. For a time he became convinced that all human behavior is determined by causes beyond the ultimate control of the individual. He felt like a helpless cork bobbing around in the ocean. Heredity set limits on his capacities. Habits and instincts bound him to predictable routines. The cure for a philosopher was more philosophy. James fortunately came across a set of essays by the philosopher Renovier. These essays made a convincing case for the concept of free will. James said that his first act of free will was to decide that he had a free will. He reported in his writings that his depression lifted, and he was able to function effectively again as a human being.

If you like, you can debate the question of free will from now to doomsday. You can construct elaborate arguments to prove that free will does not exist. You can construct equally elaborate arguments to prove that it does exist. Look in philosophy books, and you will see what I mean. But in the end you will find that the question of free will is a metaphysical question that cannot be proven once and for all either way. A metaphysical question is literally a question that is *beyond physics*. That is to say that it is beyond the real world as revealed to the human senses. Thus metaphysical questions cannot be answered by the scientific method.

All of this may sound rather elaborate and distant from the subject of weight control. But I am merely trying to convince you that you *can affirm* the existence of your free will. You may not be able to prove it on a scientific basis. But so what? Science can't prove it either. You are literally *free to be free*. If, for example, Connie G. eventually comes to feel she has free will, she will feel *above* her motives and habits. This feeling was expressed by one client as follows: "I may have a neurosis, but it doesn't have me."

WILLPOWER AND HUMAN FREEDOM

Assuming that you believe in the freedom of your own will, does this mean that you can just block your old motives and habits with willpower? Of course not. As I pointed out in the first chapter of this book, this is a misapplication of the concept of willpower. And it is the error so many overweight people make. They try to use willpower to block an impulse. The attempt is successful for a brief period. Then the dam breaks, and all good resolutions are swept away. You will recall the metaphor of the swimmer in a river presented in Chapter 1. His swimming strength was analogous to his willpower. He had the strength to *swim with the current* and out of the river to a shore. But he certainly did not have the strength to swim indefinitely upstream. But this is what so many overweight people try to do: They try to swim upstream. In a few days or weeks they are swept away by the current of temptation, and they are back to indiscriminate eating again.

Another metaphor may be of some value. Human freedom

is like the freedom of a glider returning to earth. The glider pilot is free to pick a great many landing spots *within limits*. He certainly can't decide to fly the glider to New York if he is in Southern California. Gravity and many other factors place limits on his freedom of choice. His freedom of choice, although very real, is not absolute freedom. And although he does not have absolute freedom of choice, the decisions he makes can make all the difference in the world between a crash and a safe landing.

You are like that glider pilot. You have a great deal of freedom within the constraints of your particular personality pattern. That is why an analysis of your own particular motives, defenses, and habits is so important. If you understand yourself, you can *work with* your traits. Instead of bucking yourself, cooperate with yourself. This point has been implicit throughout this book. I have said that if you are aggressive, find harmless outlets for your aggressions rather than compulsive eating. I have said that if you are an oral personality with an inordinate amount of mouth hunger, find ways of expressing this orality in nonfattening ways. But you can't completely block these impulses in yourself. Blocked, they will build up so much energy that they will burst forth and sweep away your best resolutions and all self-control. Remember this principle of cooperating with your own personality. Keep the image of the glider returning to earth in your mind. It cannot defy gravity. It must cooperate with the forces that work on it or crash. Like the adroit glider pilot, use your human freedom in a flexible way. Find ways of cooperating with your own nature.

INTERNAL CONTROL VERSUS EXTERNAL CONTROL

On the Rorschach (or inkblot) test there is a card that is often seen as two human figures facing each other. Here is

Albert Q.'s perception of the card: "This looks like two people on a merry-go-round. They're going around and around, but nobody's catching the ring." Here is Joan C.'s report: "This looks like two people dancing. They seem to be having a good time."

Remember that in a sense the inkblot *is nothing*. It is what psychologists call an ambiguous stimulus. That is to say it can be interpreted a variety of ways. The theory of the Rorschach is that the subject will psychologically structure the card in accordance with his motives and needs. The test is called a *projective test* on the general theory that a subject projects his ego outward on the blot when he gives it an interpretation. The test was devised around 1910 by Hermann Rorschach on the basis of Freudian psychoanalytic theory. Rorschach thought of the test as a way of X-raying the human personality.

The responses of Albert and Joan are very revealing. Of course, one response to one card is not enough to make a personality interpretation. But if Albert and Joan were to make a number of responses, we might see a pattern emerging. Let's assume that the responses quoted earlier were fairly typical of their responses in general. We might then have some basis for making an educated guess about their personalities. (This is just one of the scoring categories on the Rorschach that I am speaking about here. It is called *human movement.)*

It would appear that Albert does not actually see the human figures as moved from within. He sees an impersonal force moving the figures, the motor of the merry-go-round. This is very revealing in itself. It suggests that in a sense Albert feels "dead" inside. His vitality and will have left him. He is animated by external energy. Also, the merry-go-round itself is symbolical of going nowhere—going in endless circles. Finally we see that nobody's catching the ring. This conveys a sense of hopelessness and despair—human beings don't get what they want out of life. Remember, that we wouldn't want to say all of these things about Albert on the basis of one response. One response has been chosen to illustrate the concept of internal control versus external control.

On the basis of this response and other information about Albert we can say that he is a person who feels little or no internal control over his own life. He expresses the feeling that he is helpless and going nowhere.

Joan's response presents a striking contrast to Albert's. She sees two people dancing, and they are having a good time. The figures are *alive.* They are animated from within. A feeling is conveyed that life is worth living. Joan's response is a very healthy response. Taken with other tests and a psychological interview, we can say with some degree of confidence that Joan feels in charge of her own life and that life is worth living.

We could almost say that a compelling feature of common neurotic conditions is the feeling that human beings are basically nothing but marionettes, puppets manipulated by external forces. Recently I went with my family to see the famous Walt Disney film *Pinocchio.* I was a very young boy when I first saw it, but I have always remembered the movie with great pleasure. I looked forward to seeing it again in the presence of a child, and I was not disappointed. Aside from its sheer entertainment value, it struck me that one of the messages on the film is the very theme I have been discussing here. By his own efforts Pinocchio moves from being a wooden puppet to a real boy. As external control moves to internal control we find the pathway to being really alive. Certainly we have a universal theme here. Pinocchio is a symbol for every person. In order to be truly alive we must reject the feeling of being manipulated like puppets.

You can see that for Albert and Joan the freedom of the will is not a philosophical question to be debated. Perhaps they never heard of the question on an abstract basis. But they have made a choice. Albert has basically denied the existence of his human freedom. Joan has basically asserted it.

Albert is a compulsive eater. He has had a very difficult time losing weight. He feels helpless when he thinks of his weight problem. It will be necessary for him to really feel and affirm his human freedom before he can begin to lose weight. In vain he has tried everything from crash diets and pills, to hypnotists, looking for the key to his weight problem. He fails to see that all of these things are *external agents*. He is looking for the answer outside of himself. He is looking in the wrong place. As the old Al Jolson song says, "The bird with feathers of blue is waiting for you, back in your own back yard." Albert must come home to himself for the answer to his problems. Over and over again we see the wisdom of Socrates' dictum: "Know thyself." The answer lies *within*.

EXISTENTIAL-HUMANISTIC PSYCHOLOGY

The rise of scientific psychology in this century has been based to a large extent on a point of view called *behaviorism*. Behaviorism came to the general public's attention in the twenties due to the writings of its foremost spokesman in the United States, John Watson. Behaviorism stressed an objective analysis of behavior without recourse to such intangible concepts as "will," "mind," or "consciousness." In the place of such familiar concepts Watson suggested we employ the concepts of habit and the conditioned reflex. He drew enthusiastically from the works of Ivan Pavlov, the physiologist-psychologist who pioneered work on the conditioned reflex. The conditioned reflex was seen as the essential atom of human behavior. All behavior could in theory be predicted, explained, and controlled in terms of conditioning.

As a contrast to behaviorism, we have recently seen the rise of a third force in psychology. We can call this third force *existential-humanistic* psychology. It draws heavily from European existential philosophy, and from the tradition of humanism. Existential philosophy teaches that the starting point for understanding man is the *subjective* domain. The subjective domain is the inner world of the individual, and not an object of scientific scrutiny. An existential psychologist such as Rollo May, author of *Love and Will,* would say that when we describe man only in terms of his conditioning, we destroy his essential humanity. We reduce him from a person to a thing.

This point of view is stated well by another existential psychologist, Viktor Frankl, in *The Doctor and the Soul:*

> . . . the end of the nineteenth and the beginning of the twentieth century completely distorted the picture of man by stressing all the numerous restraints placed upon him, in the grip of which he is supposedly helpless. Man has been presented as constrained by biological, by psychological, by sociological factors. Inherent human freedom, which obtains in spite of all these constraints, the freedom of the spirit in spite of nature, has been overlooked. Yet it is this freedom that truly constitutes the essence of man.

Which view of man is the correct one, the behavioristic view or the existential view? It is not a question of *either-or,* of making a choice between the views. There is some truth in both views. The behaviorist approaches man from the *outside,* as an object of scientific investigation. The existential psychologist approaches man from the *inside,* as the subject of the specific and individual life he is living. The views are not opposed, but *complementary*. Rollo May, Viktor Frankl, and other existential psychologists have frequently stressed this point.

YOU ARE NOT A CONDITIONED ROBOT

What is the value of what we have been discussing for the person with an eating problem? The value is just this: You are not a conditioned robot. You are not the slave of your habits. You are not the helpless victim of unconscious motives. You are not a salivating dog. You are a human being, and you can *understand* the principles of motivation and conditioning, something a dog can never do. This understanding sets you free. Now that you have studied motivational principles and conditioning principles as they apply to eating problems, you have a powerful tool for fighting your unconscious motives and your unwanted habits.

The view I have been expounding here is as modern as twentieth-century existential psychology, and as old as ancient Greek philosophy. More than two thousand years ago Aristotle wrote about thinking. He said that man can control his impulses by the use of thought. He conceived of man as the only rational animal, the only animal that could think. And he believed that this ability to think sets man free from the bondage of primitive appetites and desires. He spoke of sensation, desire, and the reactions of an animal. Throw grain before a hungry chicken. The animal sees the grain (sensation). The sensation triggers desire. And the animal reacts by eating. But a human being can wait for an hour in a crowded restaurant and watch people eat only a few feet away without attacking their plates. Hunger may be gnawing at his stomach, but he inhibits his behavior. We have the same sensations and desires as the chicken, but unlike the chicken we can exert some control over our desires. It is dubious that you could ever teach a hungry chicken to inhibit its primitive impulses for an hour.

For the animal the formula seems to be: sensation→ desire→ a fixed reaction. For the human being Aristotle suggested the following formula: sensation→ desire→ thought→ a number of possible reactions. Thought gives the human being flexibility in his behavior. The human being has been set free by his capacity for rational reflection and thought. Throughout this book I have tried to show you the many ways that thought sets you free from the bondage of undesirable eating habits.

Your human freedom is not a philosophical question to be decided, it is something to be affirmed. There is a vast difference between the person who feels he is in the bondage of undesirable habits and the person who feels that he can alter his behavior in positive ways. A gray pall of depression seems to hang over the life of the first person. There is a sense of hopelessness about his life. Things seem out of control. The second person's life is by contrast so much brighter and better. He feels a deep sense of hope in the future, and he feels in charge of his own life. Existential psychology teaches you that you are free to make a choice.

Applying this specifically to the problem of weight control, we can say that you will lose weight and keep it off if you believe in your human freedom. Remember that you are not a programmed robot, a salivating dog, or a hungry chicken. You are a human being with the capacity to think. Use this power. *Think* and you can think yourself thin!

Chapter 12

Self-
Examination

This chapter consists of a self-examination that will help you evaluate how much you have learned from this book. The chapter is divided into two parts. Part I is the test itself. It consists of true-false questions on every chapter. These questions deal with the basic terms and concepts presented in *Think Yourself Thin*. Part II is the answer key to the test. The answer key explains briefly why each answer is either true or false.

PART I: EXAMINATION

CHAPTER 1: YOUR PROBLEM

1. In classical philosophy, the term *will* means your conscious desire.   T F

2. The right way to use willpower is in a direct confrontation with temptation.   T F

3. Psychoanalysts tend to rely upon the concepts of *unconscious motivation* and *ego defense* as explanatory principles.　　T　F

4. A large and important subfield of psychology that deals with habit formation and conditioning is called *learning theory*.　　T　F

CHAPTER 2: UNCONSCIOUS MOTIVATION

5. There is no similarity between an unconscious motive and a post-hypnotic suggestion.　　T　F

6. Overweight people seldom give superficial answers when asked, "Why do you overeat?"　　T　F

7. Feelings of inferiority, insecurity, frustration, and anxiety are manifestations of deeper problems that are often obscure, or at best half-understood.　　T　F

8. An unconscious motive is a wish or a desire that is pleasant on a conscious level.　　T　F

9. The notion that obesity can be a form of sexual defense is farfetched.

10. One way of expressing hostility toward a spouse is to become fat.　　T　F

11. The well-known cheerfulness of the overweight person is an authentic expression of his whole personality.　　T　F

12. The frustration-aggression hypothesis says that when you frustrate an organism it gets angry.　　T　F

13. Feelings of inferiority can play an important part in overeating.　　T　F

14. Involutional meloncholia is a form of mental illness characterized by great joviality.   T F

15. Overeating can be a way of avoiding people.   T F

16. Very few overweight people have anxiety about a new body image that will result when weight is lost.   T F

17. If you are suffering from unconscious motives, the situation is quite hopeless.   T F

18. One way of thinking about unconscious motives is just to say that they are motives that are obscure and half-understood.   T F

19. There is very little real danger in digging too deeply and too fast into a person's unconscious motivational structure.   T F

CHAPTER 3: OH, MY POOR EGO!

20. The ego prefers low self-esteem to high self-esteem.   T F

21. Ego defense mechanisms protect the ego in a semiautomatic fashion.   T F

22. Rationalization is a procedure by which you give yourself real reasons for your failures.   T F

23. In the ego defense mechanism called projection, the subject places blame outside himself.   T F

24. Overweight persons almost never use fantasy as a form of ego defense.   T F

25. In the ego defense mechanism called *reaction formation* there is an exaggerated conscious attitude that is opposed to a repressed unconscious attitude.   T F

26. Sometimes key questions can prick the bubble of our ego defenses.   T F

CHAPTER 4: OVEREATING IS A HABIT

27. Behavior modification is another name for psychoanalysis.   T F

28. In the jargon of conditioning theory, the bell is a conditioned stimulus.   T F

29. The most unreliable of all habit-breaking methods is called *extinction*.   T F

30. The hands of a clock pointing at 12:00 P.M. can be considered conditioned stimuli.   T F

31. The desire for sugar with coffee is not an example of a conditioned reaction.   T F

32. Instrumental conditioning deals only with what is usually called involuntary behavior.   T F

33. Much so-called voluntary behavior appears to be under the control of the reinforcement principle.   T F

34. Punishment is a good way to get rid of well-established, unwanted habits.   T F

35. When applying Premack's principle, the act with the lowest probability is used to reinforce the act with the highest probability.   T F

36. To the author of this book, the goal of an unconscious motive can be conceptualized as the "target" or "payoff" or "reinforcer" for a behavioral act.   T F

CHAPTER 5: PSYCHOLOGICAL EXERCISES

37. Negative practice simply means that you consciously and deliberately practice your bad habit.   T   F

38. The psychological exercises were designed in such a manner that the overweight person could respond to food in familiar and typical ways.   T   F

39. The psychological exercises put some "static" between the stimulus (food) and the habitual response to it (eating).   T   F

40. You should always do the exercise called "eating in front of a mirror" when other people are present.   T   F

41. Overweight people are thought to be very *field-independent;* that is to say that very little of their behavior is controlled by external cues.   T   F

42. Overeaters as a group fully enjoy and experience the taste of food.   T   F

43. One of the reasons the overweight person eats rapidly is because he is guilty about eating.   T   F

44. The exercise called "set a time." is designed to aid the overeater with the problem of snacking between meals.   T   F

45. The behavioristic psychologist Edwin Guthrie used to say that if you want to break a habit, "Practice a different response to the stimulus."   T   F

46. Because overeating is a problem with unconscious emotional roots, the habit-breaking exercises discussed are superficial and of little real value.   T   F

CHAPTER 6: CREATIVE WEIGHT CONTROL

47. Most overweight people approach a weight loss program with a spirit of creativity and adventure.　　T　F

48. Keeping a diet diary will make you more conscious of your own behavior.　　T　F

49. The weight loss graph is based on the principle of work inhibition.　　T　F

50. The on-off approach does not make psychological sense.　　T　F

51. It is not wise to set subgoals when you are trying to reduce.　　T　F

52. It is a good idea to make the act of eating involve more work than it has in the past.　　T　F

53. Putting down your fork and actually *releasing it* between every bite of food is one way of building up work inhibition.　　T　F

54. The principle of *stimulus substitution* is obviously ineffective.　　T　F

CHAPTER 7: BETWEEN HUSBAND AND WIFE

55. Loving relationships should be I-it relationships.　　T　F

56. Intimacy is one of the good results of playing games.　　T　F

57. The *I* in the I-F-D syndrome stands for individuality.　　T　F

58. Autistic thinking is seeing and hearing what you want to see and hear.　　T　F

59. Engaged couples should exchange views on serious topics before marriage. T F

60. A "game" may be defined as a set of flexible transactions in which the players make their motives known to each other. T F

61. The purpose of many marriage games is aggression. T F

62. The one who plays Jack Sprat has a need for *self-abasement*. T F

63. The one who plays the part of watchdog in the game of *Watched Dog* may have an authoritarian personality. T F

64. A watched dog overeats as a way of feeling free from the power of the watchdog. T F

65. The need operating in the one playing the part of the little boy in *Mommy's Little Boy* is a need to comply. T F

66. The yo-yo in the game called *Yo-Yo* may have a need to punish the marriage partner. T F

67. If one person refuses to play a game, this usually results in an encounter or a confrontation. T F

68. The idea of the poem "A Poison Tree" by William Blake is that it is best to contain anger. T F

69. It is wise to keep complaints general. T F

70. When another person makes you angry, it is better to describe the other person's character than to describe your inner feeling. T F

71. The idea that there can be a connection between sexual communication and overeating is very farfetched.   T   F

CHAPTER 8: HOW TO HELP A LOVED ONE LOSE WEIGHT

72. If you are overweight yourself, it is unlikely that you have a loved one who is also overweight.   T   F

73. It is a good idea for a wife to be a watchdog over her husband's eating behavior.   T   F

74. It is a good idea to praise every time you think that a word of praise is in order.   T   F

75. The double standard still prevails. Psychologically, most women are "giving" during sex and most men are "taking."   T   F

76. It is a good strategy for a husband to tease his wife about her weight.   T   F

77. The parents of overweight children are in danger of overreacting and making the problem worse.   T   F

78. It is wise to be an authoritarian and tell a child what to do about a weight problem.   T   F

79. Basically, being overweight is a child's problem, not the problem of the parents.   T   F

80. The wish to play the part of Pygmalion is a sound basis for a relationship.   T   F

CHAPTER 9: CAN PSYCHOTHERAPY HELP?

81. Most of the psychologists and psychiatrists in private practice today are pure Freudians.   T   F

82. One of the classical methods for ferreting out unconscious motives and unconscious conflicts is the method Freud called *free association*. T F

83. Hypnosis is almost a magic treatment that will make your weight problem vanish. T F

84. *Aversive conditioning* is a form of classical conditioning in which a pleasant stimulus is associated with an unpleasant stimulus. T F

85. An association of tacos with snails was an example of aversive conditioning in the chapter on psychotherapy. T F

86. In a sense many overweight persons have a kind of phobia about being thin. T F

87. In the desensitization technique, the client is instructed never to think about what he fears. T F

88. One of the advantages of group psychotherapy over individual psychotherapy is that your problems can be brought to the group for a quick solution. T F

CHAPTER 10: ANSWERS TO FREQUENTLY ASKED QUESTIONS

89. All overweight people are neurotic. T F

90. Hitting a punching bag is an example of a harmless outlet for your aggressions. T F

91. The author of this book believes that appetite depressants are very helpful in the long-run for the control of overeating. T F

92. One of the troubles with the crash diet is that it puts you into a state of suspended psychological animation. T F

93. Overweight people suffer from a lack of character.   T   F

94. Overweight people are often laughed at because they are unconsciously hated.   T   F

95. The worst kind of a snack is a high-protein snack. A snack should have sugar for quick energy.   T   F

96. Some "foodaholics" can abstain entirely from food every other day more readily than they can eat in moderation every day.   T   F

CHAPTER 11: HUMAN FREEDOM AND WEIGHT CONTROL

97. To say that you are caught helplessly in a web of habits is a very accurate statement.   T   F

98. Human freedom means the freedom to make real choices within limits.   T   F

99. Aristotle believed that thought sets you free.   T   F

100. A sense of being controlled by external agents is associated with a feeling of being fully alive.   T   F

PART II: ANSWER KEY

1. *True.* In classical philosophy, the term *will* means your conscious desires.

2. *False.* It is unwise to use willpower in a direct confrontation with temptation. You must learn how to "go with" temptation.

3. *True.* The concepts of unconscious motivation and ego defense are key concepts in psychoanalysis.

4. *True.* Learning theory is a precise investigation of habit formation and conditioning.

5. *False.* An unconscious motive and a post-hypnotic suggestion operate in similar ways.

6. *False.* Overweight people often give superficial answers when asked, "Why do you overeat?"

7. *True.* Inferiority, insecurity, frustration and anxiety are in themselves just words. The real question is *why* do you feel inferior, insecure, frustrated, and anxious?

8. *False.* An unconscious motive is a wish or a desire that is unpleasant. That is why it is unconscious.

9. *False.* It is not farfetched to think of obesity in some cases as a form of sexual defense.

10. *True.* You can express hostility toward a spouse by becoming fat. This is a form of passive-aggressive behavior.

11. *False.* Overweight people may act cheerful as a cover for underlying depression.

12. *True.* A frustrated human being is usually an angry human being.

13. *True.* Some overeating may be a form of compensation for feelings of inferiority.

14. *False.* The involutional meloncholic is depressed, not jovial.

15. *True.* One of the "payoffs" of being fat is that it may be a way of avoiding people.

16. *False.* Adjustment to a new body image is one of the problems people have to face when they lose weight.

17. *False.* Just because unconscious motives exist does not mean they cannot be made conscious. There are many ways to become more aware of your deeper motives.

18. *True.* An unconscious motive is obscure and half-understood.

19. *False.* Untrained persons should not use deep-probing techniques to dig too rapidly into unconscious motives.

20. *False.* In general, the ego prefers high self-esteem to low self-esteem.

21. *True.* Ego defenses "kick in" without your consciously willing them to do so.

22. *False.* When you rationalize, you excuse yourself. You give yourself "good reasons" instead of real reasons.

23. *True.* When you project, you blame other people or other things for your behavior.

24. *False.* Overweight persons frequently use fantasy as a form of escape from harsh reality.

25. *True.* A person using the defense called *reaction formation* demonstrates so much zeal that it is not convincing.

26. *True.* When we are using ego defense mechanisms in a maladaptive way, sometimes a question such as "Am I rationalizing?" can prick the bubble of the defense.

27. *False.* Behavior modification and psychoanalysis are both types of psychotherapy, but they are not the same approach to psychotherapy.

28. *True.* A bell is a conditioned stimulus because an organism *learns* to salivate to a bell. It is not a natural response.

29. *False.* The most reliable of all habit-breaking methods is called extinction. When a habit is not reinforced, it extinguishes of its own accord.

30. *True.* The hands of a clock pointing at 12:00 P.M. can be considered conditioned stimuli because the sight of the hands can trigger involuntary hunger reactions.

31. *False.* The desire for sugar with coffee is another example of a conditioned reaction. We *learn* to prefer coffee with sugar. We can unlearn the preference.

32. *False.* Instrumental conditioning deals with voluntary behavior, the behavior we usually think of as controlled by the will.

33. *True.* To some extent, our voluntary behavior is shaped by its own consequences. Reinforcements or "payoffs" exert their control over how we act.

34. *False.* The role of punishment in getting rid of habits is controversial. But all in all it appears that usually punishment merely has a temporarily suppressing effect on a bad habit.

35. *False.* When you apply Premack's principle, you should use the act with the highest probability as a reinforcer for the act with the lowest probability. The low-probability act should come first in time, followed by the high-probability act. This is an important principle in the art and science of self-control.

36. *True.* The goal of an unconscious motive can be conceptualized as the "target" or "payoff" or "reinforcer" for a behavioral act.

37. *True.* When you engage in negative practice, you practice your errors or your bad habits.

38. *False.* The psychological exercises were designed so that you could have the experience of responding to food in unfamiliar and unusual ways.

39. *True.* The psychological exercises are valuable because they interfere with the smooth operation of familiar eating habits.

40. *False.* In general, I recommend that the psychological exercises be done in private.

41. *False.* There is some evidence that overweight people tend to be field-dependent or very controlled by external cues. That is why the psychological exercises are so important. They help to break down the cue value of food.

42. *False.* As a group, overeaters eat so rapidly that they do not enjoy and experience the taste of food.

43. *True.* Many overweight people eat rapidly partly because they are guilty. By eating fast, they are only half-aware of how much they are eating.

44. *True.* Setting a timer and building up a self-imposed time delay is one way of learning to deal with the problem of between-meal snacks.

45. *True.* Practicing a different response to a stimulus that gives you trouble is one way of breaking bad habits.

46. *False.* Although overeating often has unconscious emotional roots, it is also important to work on your habits.

47. *False.* Most overweight people fall into the doldrums when they try to lose weight. A spirit of creativity and adventure is needed.

48. *True.* It's a good idea to keep a diet diary. It will make

you more conscious of your own behavior, an important aspect of self-control.

49. *False*. The weight loss graph is based on the principle of feedback or knowledge of results.

50. *False*. The on-off approach does make good psychological sense. It is congruent with the well-established learning principle that distributed practice is usually better than massed practice.

51. *False*. It is a very good idea to set subgoals when you are trying to reduce. You will feel more motivated to attain a goal that is close at hand.

52. *True*. Make the act of eating involve more work. This is the principle of work inhibition. It slows down the habit.

53. *True*. Putting down your fork and actually *releasing it* between every bite of food is an example of how you can use the work inhibition principle.

54. *False*. Stimulus substitution is a good idea. Try to satisfy your mouth hunger with low-calorie or high-protein snacks.

55. *False*. Loving relationships should be I-thou relationships.

56. *False*. Playing games leads *away* from intimacy.

57. *False*. The *I* in the I-F-D syndrome stands for idealization.

58. *True*. Autistic thinking is seeing and hearing what you want to see and hear.

59. *True*. Engaged couples should exchange views on serious topics before marriage. This reduces idealization to

some degree, but it creates a better understanding between people.

60. *False*. The transactions in a game are rigid and predictable. Also, the motives of the players are obscure and on a more or less unconscious level.

61. *True*. Marriage games often involve concealed hostility.

62. *False*. Jack Sprat has a need to feel superior. It is Jack Sprat's wife who has a need for self-abasement.

63. *True*. An authoritarian personality may want to play the part of a watchdog.

64. *True*. A watched dog may eat behind a watchdog's back as a way of striking a blow for personal freedom. It is a way of saying "I am free" when the watched dog does not have the courage to confront the watchdog with his feelings of oppression.

65. *True*. The husband playing the part of a little boy in the game called *Mommy's Little Boy* probably has a strong need to comply with his wife's wishes.

66. *True*. Going up and down in weight like a yo-yo is one way of punishing a marriage partner.

67. *True*. When people stop playing games, they must run the risks inherent in a confrontation or encounter.

68. *False*. In the poem "A Poison Tree" by William Blake, the idea is expressed that you will come to hate a person if you do not speak of your anger to the person.

69. *False*. Complaints should be specific. Then you argue about something concrete, not a vague abstraction. Also, you can avoid attacking the other person's character when the complaint is specific.

70. *False.* When another person makes you angry, it is better to describe your inner feelings than to describe the other person's character. This is the concept of an I-message as opposed to a you-message.

71. *False.* Sexual frustration can be one of the factors contributing to an eating problem.

72. *False.* Obesity tends to run in families.

73. *False.* It is a very poor idea for a wife to be a watchdog over her husband's eating behavior.

74. *False.* Praise should be used, but it should be used on a selective basis. Praising every time that praise seems in order soon makes the praise lose its value.

75. *True.* The concept of "give" and "take" in sex is still a widespread feeling. The woman "gives" and the man "takes." You may argue with the validity of this view. But the underlying emotional feeling is nonetheless there in most sexual exchanges between a man and a woman.

76. *False.* Teasing is a form of veiled hostility. It seldom is successful in motivating another person.

77. *True.* An overreaction to a child's weight problem often creates a long-lasting war over the issue of weight. The parent is "the enemy," and the child resists losing weight in countless ways.

78. *False.* Be an authority, not an authoritarian. An authority gives correct information and real help. An authoritarian takes over and tells someone else what to do.

79. *True.* Being overweight is at the most fundamental level the child's problem. This is very hard for some parents

to accept. But reread the discussion of this point in Chapter 8, and see if you do not find yourself finally agreeing.

80. *False.* The wish to play the part of Pygmalion is a wish to play the part of a god. It is a very unsound basis for a relationship. You will almost certainly fail in your efforts.

81. *False.* There are very few pure Freudians in private practice. Most psychologists and psychiatrists are *eclectic,* meaning they draw from many points of view in psychology.

82. *True.* Free association is one method for getting at unconscious contents.

83. *False.* Hypnosis is not a magic treatment. It may be a helpful tool in a weight control program, but the real work is still up to the overweight client.

84. *True.* In aversive conditioning, a pleasant stimulus is associated with an unpleasant stimulus.

85. *True.* An association of tacos with snails was one example given of aversive conditioning.

86. *True.* A phobia is an irrational fear. Many overweight people avoid being thin because it triggers dormant fears. These dormant fears seldom have a basis in reality.

87. *False.* In order for desensitization to take place, it is essential for the client to think about what he fears.

88. *False.* Groups do not solve problems for you. Members of a group exchange views, air feelings, and learn to evaluate their behavior on a more realistic level.

89. *False.* There is a widespread view that all overweight

people are neurotic. There is no clear and convincing evidence that this is so.

90. *True.* Hitting a punching bag is one way of discharging tension when you are angry.

91. *False.* It is my view that appetite depressants may be helpful in the short run. But in the long run, I doubt that they are of much value.

92. *True.* A crash diet puts you into a state of suspended psychological animation. When you "come out" of the state, you are likely to go back to your old eating patterns.

93. *False.* Lack of character is a descriptive phrase with little real meaning.

94. *True.* Overweight people are unconsciously hated by many people of normal weight. For this reason, overweight people are often the butt of jokes or slapstick comedy. The concealed hostility may make it difficult to make friends, get promoted, and so forth.

95. *False.* A high-protein snack is usually better than a snack high in sugar or starch.

96. *True.* A "foodaholic" can often abstain entirely from food more readily than eat in moderation.

97. *False.* To say that you are caught helplessly in a web of habits is one more rationalization.

98. *True.* Human freedom is not absolute freedom. But we can make real choices within limits.

99. *True.* The idea that thought sets you free is as old as Aristotle. He spoke clearly of this in his writings.

100. *False.* A feeling of being fully alive is associated with a sense of having internal control over your own life and destiny.

SCORING

Give yourself one point for each correct answer. Evaluate your score as follows:

> 91-100 = *Excellent.*
> 81- 90 = *Good.*
> 71- 80 = *Fair.*
> 61- 70 = *Barely passing.*
> 51- 60 = *Failure.*

I hope you received an above average score. If you did not, don't be discouraged. Read carefully the explanations that go with each question. Review the related material in the book. Repetition is often the key to complete understanding.

Assuming you are pleased with your score, I congratulate you on your success. You should feel encouraged to act on the new knowledge you have acquired. You grasped the basic concepts and terms in the book. You are armed with the fundamental understanding required to think yourself thin.

A FINAL WORD

The existential psychiatrist Viktor Frankl tells of a psychiatrist who is speaking to an alcoholic. The therapist is attempting to convince the alcoholic that he should give up his destructive drinking habit.

The alcoholic looks sadly at the psychiatrist and says, "It's too late."

The psychiatrist is thinking in positive terms. "It's *never* too late!" he insists.

The alcoholic's face brightens. "Oh! In that case I'll quit some other time!"

The alcoholic's statement has a certain logic to it. But nonetheless we recognize it as absurd. He will certainly never get anywhere with that kind of reasoning. A great rabbi said that one of the key existential questions is, "If not now, when?" Again, an affirmation is required. You must affirm that the time is *now*.

You must act on the knowledge you have acquired from this book for the knowledge to do any good. Remember that thought and action go hand in hand. You cannot think yourself thin unless you act. So act today, and start now to *think yourself thin!*

SELECTED REFERENCES

The following books and articles all deal specifically with the psychology of weight control. They are a rich source for the reader who wants to do research on the psychological factors involved in common overweight conditions. Most of the journals cited are not available in the average local library. However, Most large university libraries will have many of the journals listed. Also, your local reference librarian can usually obtain a photocopy of an article for you from a university library for a modest charge. Thus, although some of the references may seem obscure, you will not in fact find them difficult to obtain.

Berlin, I. N., Boatman, Maleta J., Sheirno, S. L., and Szurek, S. A. Adolescent alternation of anorexia and obesity. *American Journal of Orthopsychiatry*, 1951, 21, 387-419.

Brodie, Earl I. A hypnotherapeutic approach to obesity. *American Journal of Clinical Hypnosis*, 1964, 6, (3), 211-215.

Burchinal, Lee G., and Eppright, Ercel S. Test of the Psychogenic theory of obesity for a sample of rural girls. *American Journal Clinical Nutrition.*, 1959, 7, 288-294.

Bychowski, Bustav. On neurotic obesity. *Psychoanalytic Review,* 1950, 37, 301-319.

Chapman, A. L. (Public Health Service, Washington, D.C.) An experiment with group conferences for weight reduction. *Public Health Reports,* 1953, 68, 439-440.

Gluckman, M. L., et al. The response of obese patients to weight reduction. *Psychosomatic Medicine*, 1968, 30, (4), 359-373.

Gottesfeld, H. Body and self-cathexis of superobese patients. *Journal of Psychosomatic Research*, 1962, 6 (3), 177-183.

Hoebel, Bartley G., and Teitelbaum, Philip. Weight regulation in normal and hypothalamic hyperphagic rats. *Journal of Comparative and Physiological Psychology*, 1966, 61 (2), 189-193.

Hughes, Rosalie, and Reuder, Mary E. Estimate of psychological time among obese and nonobese women. *Journal of Psychology*, 1969, 70 (2), 213-219.

Karp, S. A., and Pardes, H. Psychological differentiation (field dependence in obese women) *Psychosomatic Medicine*, 1965, 27 (3), 238-244.

Kollar, E. J., and Atkinson, R. M. (Department of Psychiatry, University of California, Los Angeles). Responses of extremely obese patients to starvation. *Psychosomatic Medicine*, 1966, 28 (3), 227-246.

Kotkov, Benjamin. Experiences in group psychotherapy with the obese. *Psychosomatic Medicine*, 1953, 15, 243-251.

Lindler, Robert. "Solitaire," the story of Laura. *The Fifty Minute Hour*. Holt, Rinehart, and Winston, 1955.

Mayer, Jean. *Overweight*, Prentice-Hall, Inc., 1968.

———. Appetite and Obesity. *Atlantic Monthly*, 1955, 196, 58-62.

Rasiovsky, A., et al. Basic psychic structure of the obese. *International Journal of Psycho-Analysis*, 1950, 31, 144-149.

Rubin, Theodore. *Forever Thin,* Bernard Geis Associates, 1970.

——. *The Thin Book by the Formerly Fat Psychiatrist.* Essandess Special Editions, a division of Simon and Schuster, Inc., 1966.

Schacter, Stanley, et al. Effects of fear, food deprivation, and obesity on eating. *Journal of Personality and Social Psychology,* 1968, 10 (2), 91-97.

Silverstone, J. T., and Soloman, T. Psychiatric and somatic factors in the treatment of obesity. *Journal of Psychosomatic Research,* 1965, 9 (3), 249-255.

——. and Lascelles, B. D. Dieting and Depression: an assessment of affective disturbance occurring during clinical trial of a new anorectic preparation. *British Journal of Psychiatry,* 1966, 112 (486), 513-519.

Stuart, Harold C. Obesity in childhood. *Quarterly Review of Pediatrics,* 1955, 10, 131-145.

Stunkard, A. J. Eating patterns and obesity. *Psychiatric Quarterly,* 1959 (April), 33, 284-295.

——. The "dieting depression": untoward responses to weight reduction regimens among certain obese women. *Journal of Nervous and Mental Diseases,* 1956, 123, 194.

Sussman, Marvin B. Psycho-social correlates of obesity: failure of "calorie collectors." *Journal of the American Dietetic Association,* 1956, 32, 423-428.